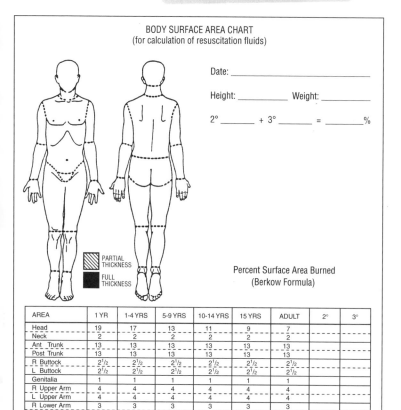

BODY SURFACE AREA CHART
(for calculation of resuscitation fluids)

Date: _____

Height: _____ Weight: _____

2° _____ + 3° _____ = _____%

PARTIAL
THICKNESS

FULL
THICKNESS

Percent Surface Area Burned
(Berkow Formula)

AREA	1 YR	1-4 YRS	5-9 YRS	10-14 YRS	15 YRS	ADULT	2°	3°
Head	19	17	13	11	9	7		
Neck	2	2	2	2	2	2		
Ant. Trunk	13	13	13	13	13	13		
Post Trunk	13	13	13	13	13	13		
R. Buttock	$2^1/_2$	$2^1/_2$	$2^1/_2$	$2^1/_2$	$2^1/_2$	$2^1/_2$		
L. Buttock	$2^1/_2$	$2^1/_2$	$2^1/_2$	$2^1/_2$	$2^1/_2$	$2^1/_2$		
Genitalia	1	1	1	1	1	1		
R. Upper Arm	4	4	4	4	4	4		
L. Upper Arm	4	4	4	4	4	4		
R. Lower Arm	3	3	3	3	3	3		
L. Lower Arm	3	3	3	3	3	3		
R. Hand	$2^1/_2$	$2^1/_2$	$2^1/_2$	$2^1/_2$	$2^1/_2$	$2^1/_2$		
L. Hand	$2^1/_2$	$2^1/_2$	$2^1/_2$	$2^1/_2$	$2^1/_2$	$2^1/_2$		
R. Thigh	$5^1/_2$	$6^1/_2$	8	$8^1/_2$	9	$9^1/_2$		
L. Thigh	$5^1/_2$	$6^1/_2$	8	$8^1/_2$	9	$9^1/_2$		
R. Leg	5	5	$5^1/_2$	6	$6^1/_2$	7		
L. Leg	5	5	$5^1/_2$	6	$6^1/_2$	7		
R. Foot	$3^1/_2$	$3^1/_2$	$3^1/_2$	$3^1/_2$	$3^1/_2$	$3^1/_2$		
L. Foot	$3^1/_2$	$3^1/_2$	$3^1/_2$	$3^1/_2$	$3^1/_2$	$3^1/_2$		
TOTAL								

Adapted from Berkow SG. A method of estimating the extensiveness of lesions (burns and scalds) based on surface area proportions. Arch Surg 8:138-148, 1924; and Lund CC, Browder NC. The estimation of areas of burns. Surg Gynecol Obstet 79:352-358, 1944.

To the memory of my mother,
Carol Ann Roth, RN

J.J.R.

■ ■ ■

To my wife, *Michelle*,
and my sons, *Liam* and *Kevin*

W.B.H.

Preface

The Philadelphia Burn Unit, located in Temple University Hospital, has dedicated its services to the care of injured patients since 1974. Inpatient admissions average 200 per year, with 2700 outpatient visits annually. *The Essential Burn Unit Handbook* is based on treatments that have evolved over a period of years and are at this time the standard of care at the burn center.

As residents serving in the Philadelphia Burn Unit, we were blessed with an experienced nursing staff, established protocols that were tempered with experience, and attending surgeons who understood the plight of the house officer. They taught us well, and they gave us the necessary latitude to mature, gain confidence, and test our mettle.

Yet we felt there had to be a better way to obtain the essential knowledge base quickly. We tried various textbooks, but we could not find concise answers to urgent issues in any one source, and the information we did find was not portable to the ER, OR, burn unit, rehab unit, trauma bay, clinic, or ward. We have been in the situation in which *you alone* have to make decisions about the management of your patient, where you must do the best you can with the tools available to you. It became clear to us that the oral tradition in which the chief resident imparts knowledge, experience, and pearls needed to be written down for the benefit of junior house officers, students, and everyone on the burn team.

This handbook represents our effort to fill a void and to communicate the common practices and workings of an active burn unit, with the rationales behind them and sample protocols to guide treatment. Our goal is to enhance the educational experience of the house officer rotating through the burn unit so that he or she can concentrate on care of the patient.

The book covers the spectrum of burn care, from initial assessment and treatment to long-term sequelae. We have included a wealth of topics that surgical residents, emergency medicine residents, and critical care fellows will encounter. These include nutrition, antibiotics, wound care, and some of the unique pathologic conditions seen in this unique and often critically injured patient population. There is content on inhalation injury and electrical and chemical burns, as well as pediatric patient management. Health care personnel involved in the care of burn patients, such as dietitians, occupational therapists, physical therapists, nurses, EMTs, respiratory therapists, and medical and nursing students, will benefit from reading this book. The handbook also includes sample orders and templates for patient presentation and organization of notes. A glossary is provided for quick reference to the many acronyms and abbreviations used in this setting.

It is our hope that this book will help the resident to provide better patient care and will shorten the resident's learning curve. This concise, pocket-sized manual goes beyond the popular "on call" and "secrets" book series, presenting more of the day-to-day management modalities than the surgical house officer books.

The treatment of burn patients is constantly evolving, and new techniques and modalities are being evaluated continually. Each patient represents a unique challenge, and therapy must be planned and tailored to the individual patient from the time of admission. Some protocols may vary from hospital to hospital—as in all of medicine, there may be more than one way to do things—but it is important to recognize that the principles remain the same.

Acknowledgments

We would like to acknowledge the contributions to this book of Dr. Frederick A. DeClement, Jr., Director of the Philadelphia Burn Unit, Emeritus, who has more than 25 years of experience in the care of burned patients. He has been our professor, mentor, and friend.

We would like to thank those who trained us, those who supported us during our training, and those who continue to support us daily as we attempt to apply what we have learned to our patients' care.

We would also like to thank the team at Quality Medical Publishing, particularly Karen Berger, Suzanne Wakefield, and Susan Trail, for helping to make this book a reality.

■   ■   ■

The Essential Burn Unit Handbook has been used by the residents in our programs. They are enthusiastic about the book and say that it has made their job easier; they particularly cite the clear explanations. We have incorporated many of their suggestions into this edition.

For such residents this book was written—for the ones called to a patient's bedside at 2 AM. If this book in some small way helps you, and in turn helps your patient, then we have accomplished what we set out to do, and our efforts have been worthwhile.

Please contact us with your questions, comments, and suggestions. We look forward to hearing from you.

Jeffrey J. Roth
William B. Hughes

Contents

1 ▪ Introduction to the Burn Unit. 1

2 ▪ Pathophysiology 3

3 ▪ Evaluation, Resuscitation, and Treatment 10

4 ▪ Wound Care, Use of Antibiotics, and Control of
Burn Wound Sepsis 42

5 ▪ Nutrition 54

6 ▪ Inhalation Injury 70

7 ▪ General (Nonburn) Inpatient Wound Care 85

8 ▪ Toxic Epidermal Necrolysis Syndrome 99

9 ▪ Electrical Burns 104

10 ▪ Chemical Burns. 108

11 ▪ Pediatric Burn Management 115

Glossary 134

Appendix. 137

Index. 139

1 ▪ Introduction to the Burn Unit

A burn patient is a unique challenge for the clinician. A burn is a common injury that represents a significant medical, social, and economic problem. Each year there are an estimated 1.2 million burn injuries and 4500 burn-related deaths in the United States.[1-3] This represents a decrease of 50% from the previous decade. Seven hundred thousand emergency room visits are made annually for burn injury. (Burn center hospitals average 200 burn admissions per year; other hospitals average fewer than five.[4]) There are an estimated 45,000 hospitalizations per year for burn injuries, about half admitted to 125 specialized burn treatment centers and half to the nation's 5000 other hospitals.[5,6]

Total hospitalizations resulting from acute burn injuries have declined 50% since 1971. Burn center admissions, meanwhile, have doubled, increasing their share from 13% to 50% of all burn patients. In the United States and Canada, there are 159 burn care centers, with more than 1900 beds.[7] The economic impact is significant: a burn of 30% of total body area can cost $200,000 for initial hospitalization costs and physicians' fees. For extensive burns, there are additional significant costs, including repeat admissions for reconstruction and rehabilitation.[8] These injuries cost the United States more than $18 billion per year.[9]

REFERENCES
1. Baker SP, O'Neill B, Ginsberg NJ, Li G. Fire burns and lightning. In Injury Fact Book, 2nd ed. New York: Oxford University Press, 1992, pp 161-173.
2. National Health Interview Survey (1991-1993 Data). American Burn Association Burn Incidence and Treatment in the U.S.: 2000 Fact Sheet. Philadelphia: The Association, 2000.

3. National Fire Protection Association (1997) Annual Vital and Health Statistics Reports of the National Center for Health Statistics (to 1994). American Burn Association Burn Incidence and Treatment in the U.S.: 2000 Fact Sheet. Philadelphia: The Association, 2000.

4. National Hospital Ambulatory Medical Care Survey (1992-1995 Data). American Burn Association Burn Incidence and Treatment in the U.S.: 2000 Fact Sheet. Philadelphia, The Association, 2000.

5. National Hospital Discharge Survey (1995-1998 Data). Agency for Health Care Policy and Research (1990-1993 HCUP-II Data). American Burn Association Burn Incidence and Treatment in the U.S.: 2000 Fact Sheet. Philadelphia: The Association, 2000.

6. American Burn Association 1991 Admissions Data. American Burn Association Burn Incidence and Treatment in the U.S.: 2000 Fact Sheet. Philadelphia: The Association, 2000.

7. Pruitt BA Jr, Mason AD Jr, Goodwin CW. Epidemiology of burn injury and demography of burn care facilities. Probl Gen Surg 7(2):235-251, Philadelphia, 1990.

8. Burn Statistics for 1992. The Bureau of Labor Statistics. Washington, DC: The Bureau, 1992.

9. Proclamation of National Burn Awareness Week, 2001. The President of the United States of America. Office of the Press Secretary, The White House, Washington, DC, February 7, 2001.

2 ▪ Pathophysiology

ANATOMY

The average adult skin surface area is 1.5 to 2.0 square meters; in a newborn the skin surface area is 0.2 to 0.3 square meters. The epidermis and dermis together range in thickness from 1 to 2 mm. The epidermis can be 0.05 mm thick, as in the eyelid, to 1 mm thick, as in the soles of the feet. Males generally have thicker skin than females do. In addition, the thickness peaks at age 30 to 40, and then thins.

The skin is derived from ectoderm and mesoderm. It has many important functions, such as protection, fluid/electrolyte homeostasis, and thermoregulation, as well as immunologic, sensory, and metabolic roles (e.g., vitamin D synthesis).

BURN CLASSIFICATION

Burns are classified by three degrees.

- *First degree* is limited to the epidermis and results in edema formation and pain.
- *Second degree* is divided into superficial and deep burns. Superficial burn wounds involve the epidermis and outer layer of the dermis. Generally, most of the dermal appendages (hair and glands) are spared. These wounds are painful, blisters occur, and the burns blanch with pressure. These are edematous and slippery to the touch because of proteinaceous exudate. Deep second-degree burns involve most of the dermal appendages. Hairs fall out with a gentle pull. The wounds are white, edem-

atous, blistered, and they are usually painless. Patients with deep second-degree burns may have compromised blood supply to the dermis and may sustain additional damage as a result of ischemia. This may convert a second-degree burn to a third-degree burn.

- *Third-degree* burns show disruption of all epithelial and dermal elements. The wound is depressed and nonedematous because of the lack of vascularization. These wounds have a leathery touch and can appear white, brown, or black. They are typically anesthetic. No spontaneous epithelialization occurs.[1,2]

ZONES OF BURN INJURY

The effects of heat are both temporal and quantitative. At temperatures of 104° to 111.2° F (40° to 44° C), enzymes malfunction, proteins denature, and cellular pumps fail. Above 111.2° F (44° C), the damage occurs faster than the cell's repair mechanism can function. Damage will continue even after the heat source is withdrawn, until the cooling process returns the skin to normal range.

As proteins denature, cell necrosis progresses, and proteins alter and coagulate. This is the first of three zones used to describe the burn wound. In the *zone of coagulation*, cell death is complete. It is usually the area nearest the heat source, and this area forms the eschar of the burn wound.

Below this zone is the *zone of stasis*. The cells are still viable, but circulation is impaired. As circulation is further compromised, ischemia results. Progressive vasoconstriction and thrombosis are seen; usually this correlates with the severity of the primary injury.[3] These microvascular changes may lead to increased damage. The entire zone could become necrotic, and turn to eschar if not healed.

The third zone is the *zone of hyperemia*. This area has minimal cellular injury but has predominant vasodilation, which increases blood flow. These cells usually recover.

Figure 2-1. The various depths of burn injury.

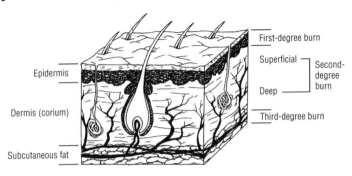

Figure 2-2. Zones of injury.

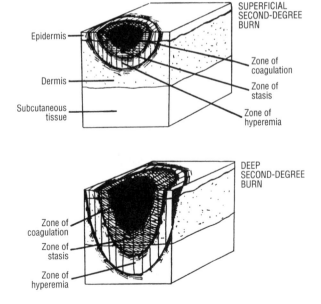

PHYSIOLOGIC RESPONSE TO BURN INJURY

Burn edema and inflammation are caused by a variety of factors. Generalized edema is usually seen in patients with burns greater than 30% total burn surface area (TBSA). The heat can directly damage vessels and increase permeability. Heat alters proteins, which activates complement, which leads to histamine release and subsequent increased vessel permeability, causing thrombosis and activation of the coagulation systems. This leads to release of serotonin (vasoconstriction) and bradykinin (increased permeability). Membrane phospholipids are altered or destroyed, which initiates the arachidonic acid cascade, leading to release of leukotrienes (increase in permeability and neutrophil recruitment), thromboxane A_2 (vasoconstriction), prostacyclin (a vasodilator), and prostaglandins (increased dilation and constriction).

These mediators as well as hypoproteinemia may also increase interstitial edema throughout the body. Microvascular injury may interfere with the function of various organ systems.[5] Dysfunction of multiple organ systems may also be secondary to neutrophils, sequestered in the lungs, liver, and other organs.[6]

Hypermetabolism is also seen with a burn injury of greater than 20% TBSA. This response can nearly double the cardiac output and metabolic rate over the next 24 to 48 hours in those patients successfully resuscitated. This hypermetabolism seems to peak at twice the normal metabolic rate in patients with burns of greater than 60% TBSA. Increased protein catabolism, increased gluconeogenesis, and insulin resistance is associated with this hypermetabolic response. This response may be secondary to a variety of factors. There may be a resetting of feedback loops, and stimulation of the hypothalamus. This results in increases in glucagon, cortisol, and catecholamines. An increase in body temperature is also stimulated.[7] The hypermetabolism can occur in response to the evaporation of heat. The response may also be influenced by a challenge to the immune system,

Figure 2-3. Physiologic response to burn.

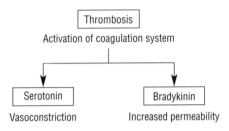

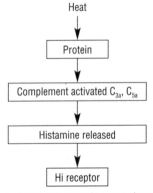

Intracellular gaps from actin-myosin contraction; protein leaks through gaps; ↑tissue colloid oncotic pressure leads to fluid shift and edema formation in connective tissue and mucosa.

Continued on p. 8.

Figure 2-3, cont'd. Physiologic response to burn.

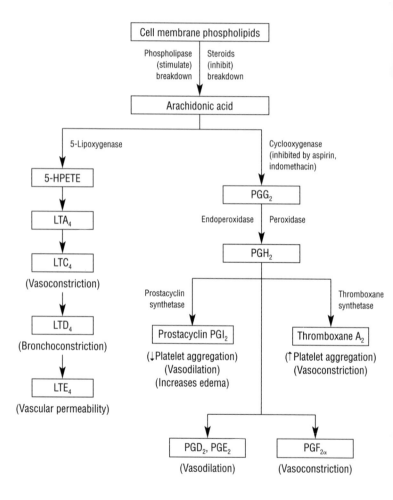

since the gastrointestinal barrier may be compromised (leading to translocation), and the lack of a normal skin barrier may serve as a portal of entry for bacteria.[8,9]

REFERENCES

1. Hinder F, Traber DL. Pathophysiology. In Herndon DN, ed. Total Burn Care. Philadelphia: WB Saunders, 1996.
2. Verheyden CN, Losee J, Miller MJ, Rockwell WB, Slezak S, eds. Plastic and Reconstructive Surgery: Essentials for Students, 6th ed. Arlington Heights, Ill: Plastic Surgery Educational Foundation, 2002.
3. Aggarwal SJ, Diller KR, Blake GK, Baxter CR. Burn induced alterations in vasoactive function of the peripheral cutaneous microcirculation. J Burn Care Rehabil 15(1):1-12, 1994.
4. Jackson DM. The diagnosis of the depth of burning. Br J Surg 40:588-596, 1953.
5. Demling R, Picard L, Campbell C, LaLonde C. Relationship of burn-induced lung lipid peroxidation of the degree of injury after smoke inhalation and a body burn. Crit Care Med 21(12):1935-1943, 1993.
6. Demling RH, LaLonde C, Liu Y, Zhu D. The lung inflammatory response from thermal injury: Relationship between physiological and histological changes. Surgery 106:52-59, 1989.
7. Youn YK, LaLonde C, Demling R. The role of mediators in the response to thermal injury. World J Surg 16(1):30-36, 1992.
8. Dietch EA. Multiple organ failure. Adv Surg 26:233-234, 1993.
9. Sasaki TM, Welch GW, Herndon DN, Kaplan JZ, Lindberg RB, Pruitt BA Jr. Burn wound manipulation-induced bacteremia. J Trauma 19(1):46-48, 1979.

3 ▪ Evaluation, Resuscitation, and Treatment

INITIAL EVALUATION

A burn patient is by definition a trauma patient. One of the main objectives of the burn unit rotation is for residents to familiarize themselves with this type of trauma, the pathophysiology, treatment modalities, and prognosis.

In short, it is important for the resident to "ignore the burn" in the initial survey, and with experience not be intimidated by the burn, but to view the patient as any trauma patient. One must follow the steps necessary to treat any trauma patient and to address the issues in the proper sequence. This principle should prevail throughout the treatment course.[1]

INITIAL RESUSCITATION
History-Taking

The first step in the diagnosis and treatment of a burn patient is to obtain a detailed history. This is extremely important. Helpful information may be obtained from the patient, witnesses, emergency personnel, and/or the fire marshal. Usually the first person to interview the patient has the best chance to document what actually happened to the patient.

The history should include the usual information, with attention given to the mechanism of injury (e.g., the patient was involved in a motor vehicle accident, an explosion, or trapped in a confined space) and the method of escape from the fire (e.g., the patient jumped from a second-story window). This will help direct the search for concomitant injuries. The agent of the burn injury is also significant (e.g., chemical, hydrofluoric acid, phosphorus, butane).

The patient's past medical history, including allergies and medications, and surgical history are also very important. Drug and alcohol history should also be noted. Documentation of these data is an essential part of history-taking. If the patient is able to communicate, one should ask the patient's height and weight. Most patients at least know this information. This is important for the calculation of body surface area, subsequent fluid rate, nutritional support, and drug dosages.

Many burns occur from attempted suicide, assault, and accidents that involve products or people. One should be aware that some form of legal action will follow in more than 50% of these cases. This is another reason that a detailed, legible history is important. The historian's name should be documented.[2]

Primary Survey

The burn should take a secondary role in the initial (primary) survey.

AIRWAY

Is the airway patent? Remember c-spine precautions.

BREATHING

Is the patient moving air?

CIRCULATION

Does the patient have a blood pressure, and is it adequate to meet the patient's metabolic needs? Is the patient bleeding?

DISABILITY

Does the patient have any gross deformities (e.g., broken bones, neurologic deficits)? Note any penetrating injuries (both front and back). Perform a neurologic examination.

EXPOSURE

Disrobe the patient and perform an examination, including a rectal examination. Place a Foley catheter for accurate measurement of input and output. Place a nasogastric tube (NGT) for stomach decompression, ulcer prophylaxis, and enteral feedings.

Secondary Survey

AIRWAY

Is the face involved as a result of flame injury? Are there any blackened or charred areas around the airway? Is there any carbonaceous sputum? Is the patient hoarse? Is stridor present? Is soot present in the oropharynx? Is the patient able to clear his or her secretions?

BREATHING

Is the patient moving a sufficient amount of air? Consider bronchoscopy to document airway damage and swelling secondary to heat, or toxins. In any inhalation injury or significant burn injury, consider intubation. This is especially important in light of the massive fluid resuscitation necessary, which may cause edema, leading to upper airway obstruction. Intubation will also protect the airway against delayed compromise resulting from injury that may not have been appreciated at the time of the initial examination. Consider escharotomy if the burns on the chest are full thickness and involve the entire anterior chest wall or if the patient is not moving adequate volumes of air. If the wounds are partial-thickness burns, consider chemical escharotomy with a proteolytic agent, such as Collagenase or Accuzyme (which functions in a broader pH range).

CIRCULATION

Monitor pressure and signs of perfusion (warm kneecaps, warm toes, adequate urine output). Secure IV access for resuscitation with suturing; do not use tape, because tape will lose its adhesive properties. Large-gauge peripheral lines are best used early in the resuscitative effort. Central access is needed for hemodynamic monitoring, drawing blood, and access for aggressive fluid resuscitation. The central access initially may be placed through the burn. This access should be sutured in four places to ensure stability. Maintenance of secure venous access is critical. In our protocol the access will be changed in 3 days to decrease the potential for line sepsis and thrombus formation.

Burn edema accelerates with fluid resuscitation, making veins difficult to visualize, palpate, and cannulate. Remove all rings, chains, and other items that may constrict the patient when edema is present.

Resolution of the edema will occur when the microvascular system and the cell membranes recover from the thermal insult and resorption of the fluid from the extravascular space begins. This diuretic or mobilization phase usually occurs on the fourth to sixth day, but may extend for longer periods.

Search for any areas of hemorrhage, look for penetrating injuries, be sure to logroll the patient and inspect, palpate, and auscultate the back and spine. Always roll the patient toward yourself; the examiner on the other side will then examine the patient. Now roll the patient the other way; your colleague will roll the patient toward himself or herself and hold the patient. You now can examine the patient. A CT scan may be necessary for evaluation.

DISABILITY

Address potential traumatic injuries. This is especially important in light of a significant mechanism of injury (e.g., auto accident, explosion, or traumatic escape). Remember to logroll the patient. Examine the patient from head to toe. Palpate over bones. Examine all areas, including between the buttocks and the perineal area. The use of adequate light will help your examination.

EXPOSURE

In the body diagram, note the areas of burn (Figs. 3-1 and 3-2). Make a drawing of the burn, noting the depth, and determine whether the burn extends across a joint or is circumferential. If the burn is circumferential, an escharotomy may be necessary. Estimate the total burned surface area (TBSA) using Berkow's percentages chart (Fig. 3-3). Another convenient way of estimating percentage of burn is to use the palmar surface of the patient's hand. The palmar surface (including the digits) can be estimated to be 1% (actually, it is 0.85%) of the body surface. Note also that the palmar surface of their hand minus the palmar area of the digits can be considered to be 0.5% BSA.[3] In calculating the TBSA, do not include first-degree burns. Record the estimated percentage of burn in the appropriate space. This estimate may change after removal of soot and dirt in the tub room. Some areas of pigmented collapsed bullae of partial-thickness injury later may be debrided with dressing changes.

RESUSCITATION

We use the Parkland formula as a starting point for fluid resuscitation. Initial fluid replacement with lactated Ringer's solution begins at 4 ml × Body weight in kilograms × % Total body surface area (%TBSA) of the burn injury (e.g., 4 ml × 70 kg × 60% burn = 16,800 ml). This can be done quickly using the "Rule of nines" (see Fig. 3-1): In an adult the head, each upper extremity, the anterior chest, posterior thorax, abdomen, and buttocks each equal approximately 9% TBSA. Each lower extremity is 18% TBSA. Note that these percentages shift for pediatric patients (see Fig. 3-2). The more accurate and preferred way to estimate TBSA is the Berkow/Lund chart (Fig. 3-3). Use Fig. 3-3 for drawing the TBSA and for calculation of resuscitation fluids. Begin calculation of fluid resuscitation from the time of injury, not when the patient arrives in the emergency room (ER). The first half of this volume is to be administered within 8 hours of the burn (even if there is a delay in getting the patient to a medical center). The second half of the volume is given over the next 16 hours. A too-rapid decrease in the fluid resuscitation may result in hypotension and/or a decrease in the urinary output. Therefore we decrease the fluid volume by 50 to 100 ml/hr until the calculated dose is achieved. Remember that the calculations are a guide. One must tailor the volume replacement to the individual patient. We use urine output as an indicator of the adequacy of fluid resuscitation. Acceptable urine output is usually 0.5 ml/kg/hr (usually 30 ml).

After the first 24 hours, the maintenance fluid is $D_5\frac{1}{2}NS$. The rate calculated for 24 hours by using the following guideline.

Method for Calculating Maintenance Fluid

First 10 kg	100 ml/kg
Second 10 kg	50 ml/kg
Every kilogram above 20 kg	20 ml/kg

For example, a 70-kg patient's calculation would be 100×10 (for the first 10 kg) + 50×10 (for the second 10 kg) + 50×20 (for the 10 other kilograms not yet covered): $1000 + 500 + 1000 = 2500$ ml/24 hr. This totals 104 ml/hr for maintenance fluids. Remember, this is an estimate and you can round up to more manageable numbers (e.g., 105 ml/hr).

During the fourth 8-hour period after a burn, salt-poor albumin (SPA) is infused using the formula $(0.1) \times$ (kilograms) $\times$ (%TBSA). Infuse the SPA over 4 to 6 hours.

Water of evaporation must be calculated at this time for those burns >25%. This equation is:

$$\%TBSA + (25 \times BSA \text{ in } m^2) =$$
Number of milliliters of evaporative water loss/hr

Text continued on p. 28.

Figure 3-1. Rule of nines: body diagram for estimation of total burned surface area (%TBSA) in adults (numbers are for anterior only and posterior only).

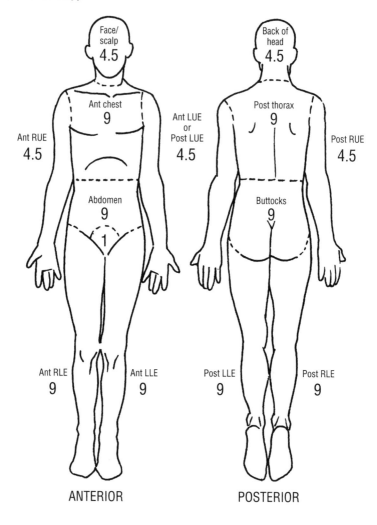

ANTERIOR   POSTERIOR

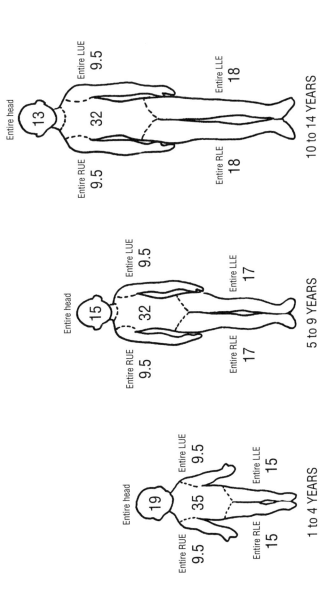

Figure 3-2. Rule of nines, modified for pediatric patients: body diagram for estimation of total burned surface area (%TBSA) in children (numbers include anterior and posterior).

Figure 3-3. Diagram and chart for estimating total burned surface area. (Adapted from Berkow SG. A method of estimating the extensiveness of lesions [burns and scalds] based on surface area proportions. Arch Surg 8:138-148, 1924; and Lund CC, Browder NC. The estimation of areas of burns. Surg Gynecol Obstet 79:352-358, 1944.)

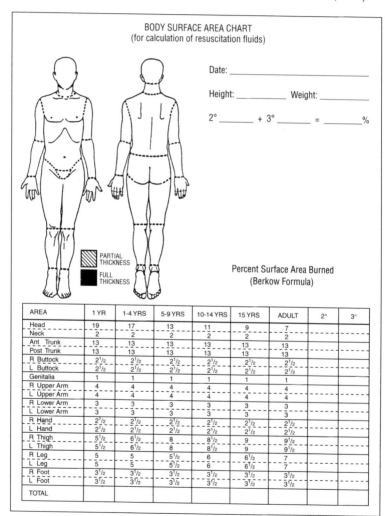

BODY SURFACE AREA CHART
(for calculation of resuscitation fluids)

Date: _____

Height: _____ Weight: _____

2° _____ + 3° _____ = _____%

PARTIAL THICKNESS

FULL THICKNESS

Percent Surface Area Burned
(Berkow Formula)

AREA	1 YR	1-4 YRS	5-9 YRS	10-14 YRS	15 YRS	ADULT	2°	3°
Head	19	17	13	11	9	7		
Neck	2	2	2	2	2	2		
Ant Trunk	13	13	13	13	13	13		
Post Trunk	13	13	13	13	13	13		
R Buttock	$2^1/_2$	$2^1/_2$	$2^1/_2$	$2^1/_2$	$2^1/_2$	$2^1/_2$		
L Buttock	$2^1/_2$	$2^1/_2$	$2^1/_2$	$2^1/_2$	$2^1/_2$	$2^1/_2$		
Genitalia	1	1	1	1	1	1		
R Upper Arm	4	4	4	4	4	4		
L Upper Arm	4	4	4	4	4	4		
R Lower Arm	3	3	3	3	3	3		
L Lower Arm	3	3	3	3	3	3		
R Hand	$2^1/_2$	$2^1/_2$	$2^1/_2$	$2^1/_2$	$2^1/_2$	$2^1/_2$		
L Hand	$2^1/_2$	$2^1/_2$	$2^1/_2$	$2^1/_2$	$2^1/_2$	$2^1/_2$		
R Thigh	$5^1/_2$	$6^1/_2$	8	$8^1/_2$	9	$9^1/_2$		
L Thigh	$5^1/_2$	$6^1/_2$	8	$8^1/_2$	9	$9^1/_2$		
R Leg	5	5	$5^1/_2$	6	$6^1/_2$	7		
L Leg	5	5	$5^1/_2$	6	$6^1/_2$	7		
R Foot	$3^1/_2$	$3^1/_2$	$3^1/_2$	$3^1/_2$	$3^1/_2$	$3^1/_2$		
L Foot	$3^1/_2$	$3^1/_2$	$3^1/_2$	$3^1/_2$	$3^1/_2$	$3^1/_2$		
TOTAL								

Figure 3-4. Escharotomy sites (whole body view).
(Adapted from Greenfield LJ, Mulholland M, Oldham KT, Zelenock GB, Lillemoe KD. Surgery, Scientific Principles and Practice, 2nd ed. Philadelphia: Lippincott-Raven, 1997.)

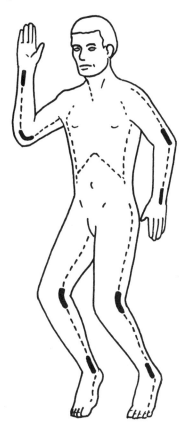

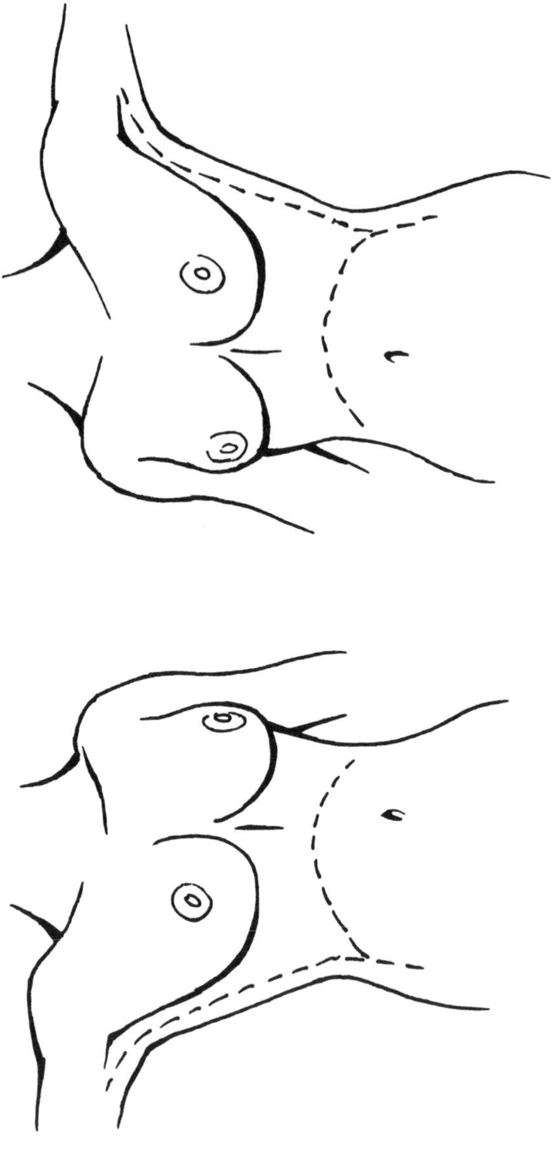

Figure 3-5. Left and right trunk. Dashed lines indicate escharotomy incisions.

Figure 3-6. Left and right hands. Dashed lines indicate escharotomy incisions.

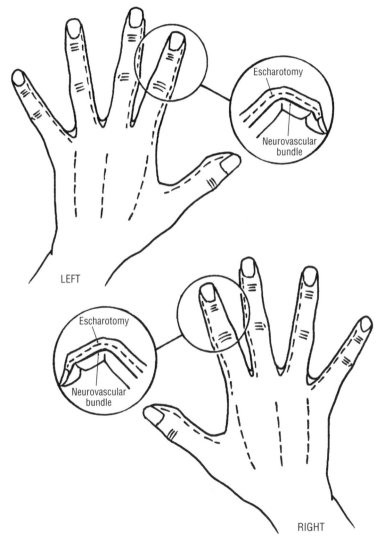

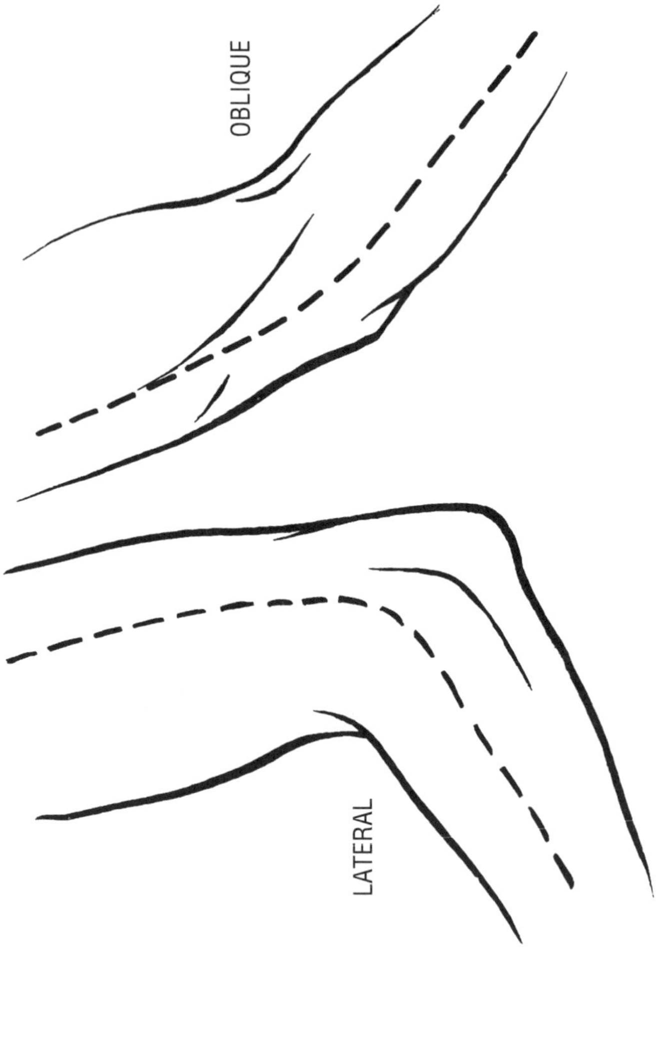

Figure 3-7. Left elbow. Dashed lines indicate escharotomy incisions.

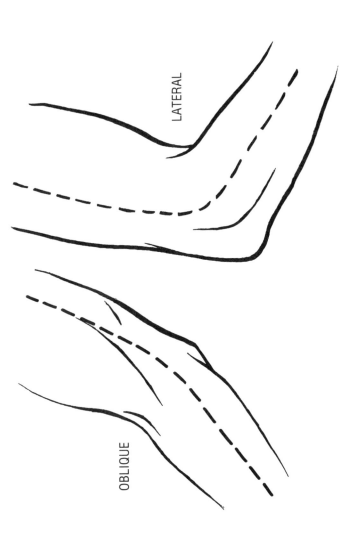

Figure 3-8. Right elbow. Dashed lines indicate escharotomy incisions.

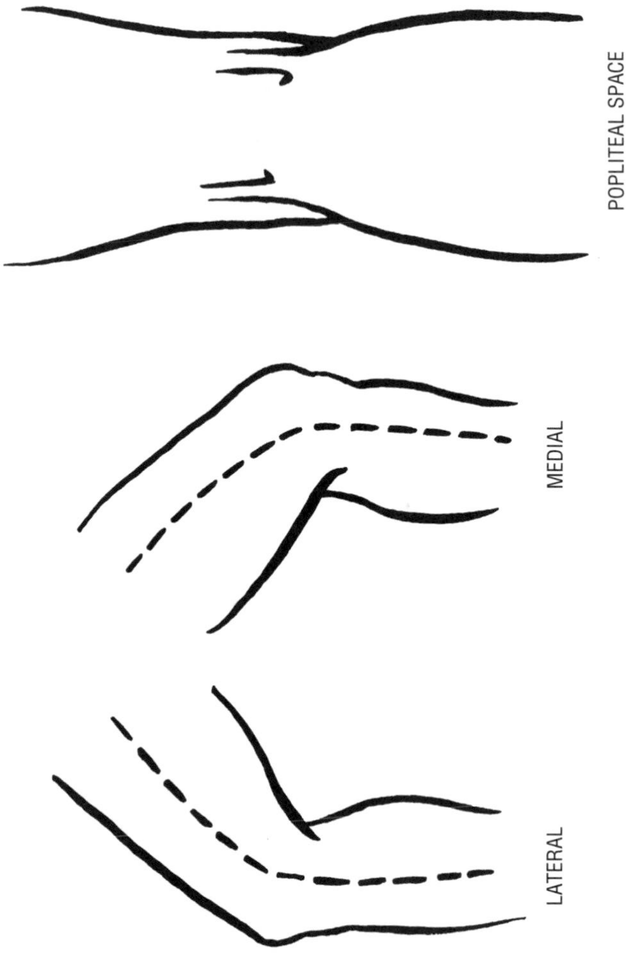

Figure 3-9. Left leg. Dashed lines indicate escharotomy incisions.

Figure 3-10. Right leg. Dashed lines indicate escharotomy incisions.

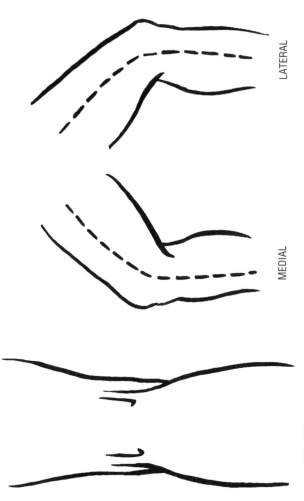

LATERAL

MEDIAL

POPLITEAL SPACE

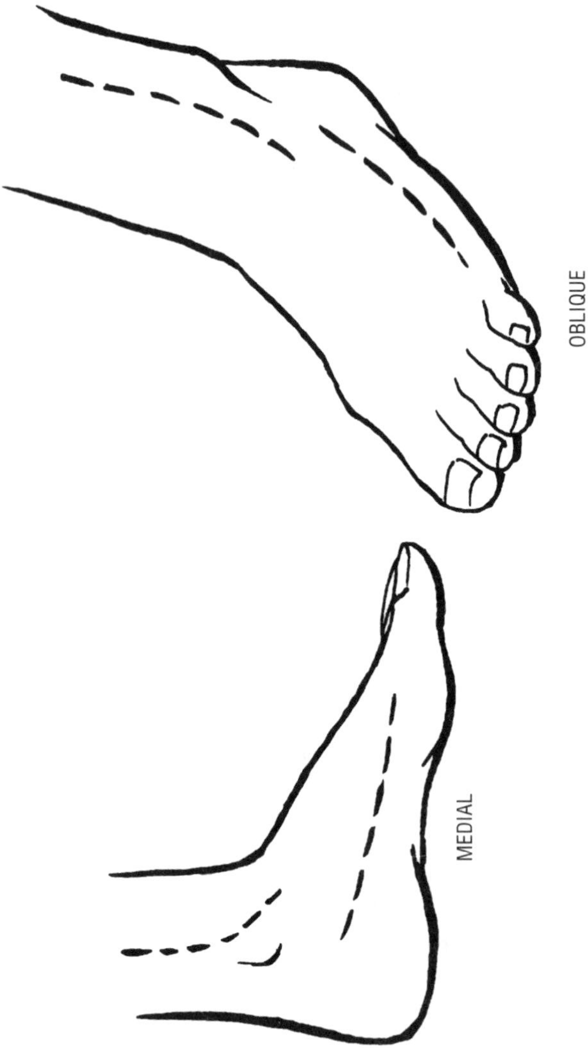

Figure 3-11. Left foot. Dashed lines indicate escharotomy incisions.

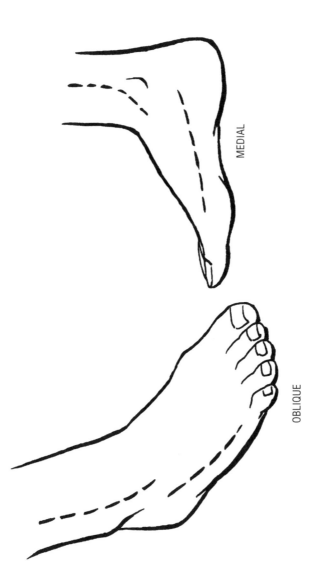

Figure 3-12. Right foot. Dashed lines indicate escharotomy incisions.

MEDIAL

OBLIQUE

Body surface area (BSA) is calculated as follows (*do not confuse with total burned surface area*):

[87 (H + W) − 2600] ÷ 10,000 = Surface in m²

H = Height in cm and W = weight in kg

Replace this amount as free water. Evaluation of serum Na will give an indication of adequate replacement. The optimal level of Na to be maintained is 135 to 137 mg/dl. As the slope of the curve of Na levels changes, trends can be determined and corrected before increased losses are present.

ASSESSMENT OF OTHER PARAMETERS

Obtain trauma laboratory values and carboxyhemaglobin and arterial blood gas levels, a chest x-ray (CXR) evaluation, and ECG.

Avoid hypothermia by wrapping the patient with warm blankets. Covering the head will conserve significant amounts of heat. Hypothermia is secondary to the patient's skin loss. This regulatory barrier is now damaged, and the patient will lose heat by convection, conduction, radiation, and evaporation. This may occur subtly in a wet, undressed, hypotensive patient, despite routine monitoring. Dressings are placed to minimize heat and water losses to a minimum and keep antibacterial creams in contact with the burn injury.

WHAT'S NEXT

The patient will undergo debridement in the burn center. This should take place in a room with warm ambient temperature (at least 82° F [28° C]). The process will be aided by immersion of the injured area in warm water. Escharotomy may be performed at this time if indicated, with electrocautery equipment; intravenous sedation is given to the patient. Escharotomy is performed on the medial and lateral surfaces of the extremities (Figs. 3-4 through 3-12), on the anterior axillary line, and subcostally on the chest (see Fig. 3-4). The incision is made down to the fat layer. In patients with little subcutaneous tissue, great care must be exercised to avoid inadvertent fasciotomy.

Large vessels injured during this process should be ligated with 4-0 ties. However, if the escharotomy is carefully performed, there should be little bleeding from the incised margins. Paradoxically, a pitfall of escharotomy is not making the incision deep enough. If there are dermal strands extending across the incision, the expansion of the tissue will be hampered.

ADMITTING A PATIENT TO THE BURN UNIT

The continuation of resuscitation, close monitoring, critical care, and wound care are best managed in a dedicated unit by personnel trained in the care of this unique patient population.

Sample Admission Orders
(Do not write comments—shown here in italics—on the order sheet.)

ADMISSION
   To burn unit

DX
   s/p trauma, 50% TBSA burn secondary to falling asleep while smoking in bed.

HEIGHT AND WEIGHT

CONDITION
   Critical

VITAL SIGNS
   Per routine. [Continuous monitoring of vitals. Record qh; call HO if temp >102.5° F (39° C), p <60 or >100, BP <100 systolic or >160 systolic, pulse ox <90. Measure strict I&O qh; notify HO if <0.5 ml/kg/hr *(usually 30 ml/hr)*]. Monitor CV; record qh.

ALLERGIES
   (Document allergies. Watch drug interactions.)

ACTIVITY

Bed rest. Head of bed at 20 degrees. *(To minimize cerebral and tracheal edema.)* No pillow for head and neck burns. *(To minimize contractures and damage to ears.)*

NURSING

Per routine. Wound care as per unit protocol. *(See Chapter 4 for examples of such a protocol.)*

DIET

NPO if burn >30%. Enteral feedings with TraumaCal or a similar formula. *(Target feedings of 25 Kcal/kg/day times 2.0 [stress factor].)*

Tube feedings:

½ strength @ 25 ml/hr × 4 hr, then
¾ strength @ 25 ml/hr × 4 hr, then
Full strength @ 25 ml/hr × 4 hr, then
Increase 15 ml/q4h to goal.
Check residuals q4h; hold if >150 ml.

IV FLUIDS

Per Parkland formula. *(Administer through large-bore catheter sutured in place.)*

4 ml LR × kg × %TBSA
Give half in the first 8-hr period.
Give half in the next 16-hr period.

(Maintain urine output at 0.5-1.0 ml/kg/hr.)

If an inhalation injury is present in adults, the alteration may need to be 5 × kilograms × %TBSA. In elderly patient or in children, the Parkland formula may need to be altered to 3 × kilograms × %TBSA.

MAINTENANCE FLUIDS

Next give $D_5\frac{1}{2}NS$ at maintenance level *(+ evaporative loss, if* **TBSA** *is >25% [% of burn] + [25 × BSA in m^2] = Milliliters of evaporative water loss/hr])*. Replace this amount as free water.

Give albumin (SPA) in the fourth 8-hr period *(0.1 × kilograms × %TBSA)*. **Note:** *SPA is a 25% solution.*

If your institution stocks only plasmanate (a 5% colloid solution), the calculation for colloid administration is 0.5 ml × kilograms × %TBSA.

MEDICATIONS

Topical antibiotics

Silver sulfadiazine (Silvadene) on body; bacitracin-polymyxin B (Polysporin) on face

Mycostatin (Nystatin) 200,000 U PO/NGT q8h *(To inhibit bacterial transorption.)*

Lactinex 1 g PO/NGT q6h

Tetanus toxoid 0.5 ml IM

Hypertet 250 U IM *(for older patient and/or if there is no history of immunization)*

Carafate 1 g PO/NGT q6h *(use for a >20% burn)*

MVI 10 ml IV qd

Folate 1 mg PO/NGT/IV qd

$MgSO_4$ 500 mg qw *(if >50% burn)*

Pain medications

Dilaudid 2 mg IV q4h

MSO_4 8 mg IV q4h

Other agents

Vitamin C 1000 mg PO/NGT/IV q6h

$ZnSO_4$ 220 mg PO/NGT tid

Selenium 50 mg PO/NGT bid

Vitamin E 400 U PO q6h

Beta-carotene 25,000 U PO q12h

Heparin 5000 U SQ q8h

Metamucil 1 Tbsp PO/NGT bid

Codeine 30 mg PO q6h prn for diarrhea

ADDITIONAL ORDERS

If the patient has an eye burn:

Gentamycin ophthalmic solution *(formulation and strength carried by your pharmacy)*

If the patient has a pulmonary injury:

Aminophyline *(6.0 mg/kg IV load, then 0.5 mg/kg/hr IV)*

Ventolin (0.5 mg in 2 ml NS via nebulizer q4h and prn)

Heparin *(4000 U [mix with Ventolin nebulizer in the 2 ml NS] will help to decrease pulmonary casts)*

(Consider bronchoscopic evaluation.)

If the patient has no pulmonary injury:

Oxygen per nasal cannula or high-humidity face mask

Chest physical therapy

If the patient has sustained electrical injury:

Complete spine series *(Be sure to visualize C7/T1.)*

Long bone x-ray film series

Urine myoglobin and hemoglobin assay

Dopamine, renal dose, 1-4 µg/kg/hr IV

If the patient is elderly (optional):

Dopamine, renal dose, 1-4 µg/kg/hr IV

EXTRA ORDERS

NGT to LCWS flush q2h with 30 ml NS

Daily weight measurement

Bed in 20-degree semi-Fowler's position

Elevate extremities

Foot cradle, splints

Abduct shoulders

Foley to gravity

Decubitus precautions

No pillow for a head/neck burn

VENTILATOR SETTINGS AND PEEP
>   Preferred ventilator: VDR_4
>> Initial settings
>>> Ausculatory rate 600
>>> PIP 30-35
>>> 2-sec inspiration
>>> 2-sec expiration

(If your institution does not have this equipment available, use these standard settings. For nonburn patients, usually start on AC-10, V_T of 10-15 ml/kg, 100% FIo_2, 5 PEEP. Burn patients require increased respiratory rate and decreased tidal volume, because contraction from the burn limits chest expansion. Therefore start at AC 15-20, V_T 5-10 ml/kg. Check an ABG in 30 min and make adjustments accordingly.)

>   Obtain an ABG 30 min after the patient is placed on the ventilator *(And make changes accordingly.)*
>   ABG/carboxyhemoglobin *(Obtain on admission and prn.)*
>   ECG *(Obtain on admission and prn.)*
>   CXR *(Obtain on admission; we usually obtain one on M and F, and prn. A CXR is obtained qd for patients receiving ventilatory support; assess for infiltrate, tube placement, pneumothorax.)*

LABORATORY TESTS
>   CBC *(On admission and W.)*
>   SMA-12 *(On admission and M.)*
>   SMA-7 *(On admission and M-W-F and prn.)*
>   PT/PTT *(On admission and prn.)*
>   Sputum C&S *(On admission and qd and prn.)*
>   Ca, Mg, Phos *(On admission and biweekly.)*
>   H&H/electrolytes *(q8h; do this until the patient is stable and then prn.)*
>   Finger stick blood sugar *(On admission and tid and prn.)*
>   Urine 24-hr electrolytes *(On admission.)*
>   HIV/EtOH/urine drug screen *(On admission.)*

B-HCG *(If patient is female.)*
Sickle cell panel *(If patient is black.)*
Eschar BX *(prn)*
Albumin, prealbumin, transferrin *(qw [on M].)*

CONSULTATIONS
OT/PT
Nutrition

OTHER CONSULTATIONS *(prn)*
(Consent required for HIV testing, placing central lines, grafting, blood transfusions.)

CRITICAL CARE: ORGANIZATION FOR NOTES AND PRESENTATION

SHORT HISTORY
"This is Mr. X, a 25-year-old BM post burn day 3 s/p 50% TBSA burns after falling asleep while smoking in bed. He is also post-operative day (POD) 2 from wound debridement and STSG to chest, along with application of pigskin to the remainder of the burned area."

T_{max}, INPUT/OUTPUT

NEUROLOGIC
Awake/alert, oriented ×3, GCS
Sedated, agent, rate
Paralysis, agent, rate
Focal vs. nonfocal

PULMONARY
Examination
Secretions
Ventilator settings
AC vs. SIMV vs. CPAP/rate/pressure
Spontaneous rate/VT/FIO_2/PEEP/pressure support

ABG

CXR

CV/HEMODYNAMIC

Pulse, BP, patient on any pressors (dopamine, dobutamine)

Swan-Ganz catheter parameters

PAP/wedge/CO/SVR/Svo_2 or Mvo_2

Electrolytes, anion gap, lactate

O_2 delivery, content

GI/NUTRITION

Examination

Obstruction series (if done)

Drainage output (if any)

BEE, calories needed, goal, plan to achieve that goal

[Note the location of the feeding catheter. Feedings to the stomach may increase tonicity first, followed by increased volume. Feedings to the small bowel increase volume first, then tonicity (to avoid diarrhea).]

Feedings; name, strength, rate, route, nutritional parameters, UUN *(to compute nitrogen balance)*, transferrin, prealbumin, albumin

RENAL

Urine output (ml/kg/hr); minimum required is 0.5 ml/kg/hr

BUN/Cr or FENa if the UO is low

INFECTIOUS DISEASE/SEPSIS

WBC, blood and other cultures; site of focality; antibiotics (include day number)

ENDOCRINE

Function tests; LFTs; fingersticks; steroids

HEMATOLOGY/ONCOLOGY
Hb, platelet count PT/PTT, coagulopathy studies *(if indicated)*
SMA-7

SKIN
Percentage of burn, treatments, percentage take of graft *(may be brought up earlier in burn unit presentation)*
Decubitus

EXTREMITIES
PT/OT treatment, progress

WHAT HAPPENS NEXT: THE PLAN
Debridement and Coverage

In general, one wishes to excise the nonviable tissue and cover the wound as soon as possible. Options for initial coverage include skin grafting, allograft, pigskin, CEA, Alloderm with STSG, Integra.[6] (This subject is covered in more detail in Chapter 4.)

PREOPERATIVE EVALUATION

Vital signs
Procedure, indications
Laboratory tests
Type and crossmatch or screen for PRBCs *(Obtain this at least 24 hours before surgery to allow the blood bank to obtain compatible blood when antibodies are present.)*
(Blood loss with debridement is now less of an issue since the use of epinephrine/saline solution infiltration before debridement and skin harvesting from donor sites.)
CXR, ECG
Informed consent signed and on chart
OR notified; anesthesia team notified

REPEAT EXCISIONS AND GRAFTS

The ultimate goal in dealing with a burn wound is to close it as soon as possible, allowing the skin to heal spontaneously, or using skin grafting to provide permanent coverage of the wound.

Rapid removal of the burn wound eliminates a source of tissue breakdown products, bacteria, and cytokine activation. This allows the patient to stabilize more quickly and results in a more desirable cosmetic and functional result.

Patients with large burn injuries may not have enough uninvolved skin to furnish an adequate amount of donor skin. This should not delay excision of the burn wound, because other wound coverings are available. Excised surfaces may be covered temporarily with cadaver allograft, Integra, Biobrane, or porcine xenograft (in that order of desirability). Skin biopsies may be sent to allow cultured skin growth (CEA).

SPECIAL AREAS OF BURN INJURY
Face

Burns on the face do well with daily application of bacitracin or another triple-antibiotic ointment. Patients with facial burns or a significant mechanism should have an ultraviolet light test for corneal abrasions. Ophthalmologic evaluation may be sought if indicated. Ears can be treated with mafenide only. This agent may decrease the incidence of chrondritis and helps to avoid the risk of pressure necrosis. If the ears are to be wrapped, carefully place padding behind them to avoid pressure injury.[7]

Extremities

All burned extremities should be dressed with silver sulfadiazine (Silvadene). Surginet (expandable fishnet) over 4 × 4 sterile dressings works well. The extremities should be kept elevated. Hand burns can usually be cared for on an outpatient basis. Functional, vascular, and neurologic assessment should be documented. Digits should be kept in a straight position and wrapped individually. Again, 4 × 4s with fishnet dressings work well. These patients should be seen the next day in the burn office. Close follow-up is crucial to the care of these patients. These patients benefit from early intervention of an occupational therapist.

ALLIED HEALTH PRACTITIONERS: PART OF THE TEAM

Management of the burn patient is a multidisciplinary team effort and extends from the time of injury to completion of the patient's rehabilitation—that is, possibly years. All practitioners are important members of this team.

Occupational Therapists

Occupational therapists focus on the function of the hand, involving activities of daily living, and on scar control. Modalities of therapy include splinting for immobilization and positioning as well as devices for patient mobilization and those to adapt the patient to his or her surroundings and abilities.

Physical Therapists

Physical therapists focus on the general mobility of the patient, and the mobility of the extremities. Modalities include therapy, splinting and adaptation devices. Spandex compression garments are custom fitted to the patient. They compress the burned area in an effort to flatten and soften scar tissue as it matures. Inserts are sometimes placed within the spandex pressure garments to apply more directed pressure to those areas that are difficult to address with garments alone.

Dietitians

Dietitians focus on the nutritional status of the patient, enabling him or her to compensate for the tremendous metabolic needs associated with recovery from a burn. This is a crucial issue in this patient population, because these patients need adequate substrates to heal their wounds and handle the endocrine and metabolic stresses. Dietitians can calculate the caloric requirements and monitor the patient's dietary and weight trends. They are also knowledgeable about the characteristics of the myriad enteral and perenteral formulas that may benefit the patient.[8,9]

OTHER ISSUES

In our unit, we change CVP catheters every 3 days. These catheters are not changed over a wire; the site is changed each time. We have found that this can significantly cut down on the incidence of infection and thrombosis.

Intravenous antibiotics are used, guided by culture data and clinical evaluation. Clinical evaluation is needed to assess distinctions between colonization and infection. Prophylactic antibiotic therapy is not used; this helps to prevent the appearance of more resistant organisms. Often burn patients have mild fevers secondary to their hypermetabolic state. Therefore the threshold for fever workup, culturing, and treatment is 102° F (39° C) in most cases.[10,11]

The choice of bed is covered in greater detail in Chapter 5. Generally, the goal is to decrease the amount of sheering forces. Some beds can help in pulmonary toilet, facilitating access to the patient for rotation and percussion therapy.

STEP-DOWN BURN CARE

The patient will often be sent to a general hospital unit after the critical portion of his or her hospital course has been accomplished. The intensive occupational therapy, physical therapy, and nutritional support continue.

Rehabilitation

The rehabilitation process that was started in the burn unit continues. Some patients need to go to a designated rehabilitation facility, whereas others may continue their therapy on an outpatient basis.

Preparing for Discharge to Home

The goal of therapy is to have the patient return to his or her home and occupation in the best functional condition. Modifications in the home situation are sometimes necessary. This can range from care issues to physical changes in the residence. Social workers and case managers are important resources in this aspect of care.

Psychiatric Care for a Burn Patient

A burn patient also sustains significant emotional trauma and stress. There are many issues: physical self-image, possible loss of loved ones, home, and possessions. Emotional and psychologic support is very important to the outcome, rehabilitation, and adaptation of the individual. A psychiatrist may also help the family or a significant other cope with the aftermath of a serious burn injury. There are self-help organizations and support groups for burn patients that address social, functional, and occupational concerns.[12]

Psychiatric consultation in the acute phase of burn injury is important, as is postdischarge follow-up. Members of the burn team should be alert to the fact that even relatively minor burn injuries can have a major psychologic impact on the patient and family. Do not hesitate to recommend psychiatric evaluation and support.

REFERENCES
1. Advanced Trauma Life Support, 7th ed. Chicago: American College of Surgeons, 2000.
2. Cupera J, Mannova J, Rihova H, Brychta P, Cundrle I. Quality of prehospital management of patients with burn injuries—a retrospective study. Acta Chir Plast 44(2):59-62, 2002.

3. Sheridan RL, Petras L, Basha G, Salvo P, Cifrino C, Hinson M, McCabe M, Fallon J, Tompkins RG. Planimetry study of the percent of body surface represented by the hand and palm. Sizing irregular burns is more accurately done with the palm. J Burn Care Rehab 16(6):605-606, 1995.

4. Berkow SG. A method of estimating the extensiveness of lesions (burns and scalds) based on surface area proportions. Arch Surg 8:138-148, 1924.

5. Lund CC, Browder NC. The estimation of areas of burns. Surg Gynecol Obstet 79:352-358, 1944.

6. Deitch EA. A policy of early excision and grafting in elderly burn patients shortens the hospital stay and improves survival. Burns Incl Therml Inj 12(2):109-114, 1985.

7. Stanton RA, Billmire DA. Skin resurfacing for the burned patient. Clin Plast Surg 29(1):29-51, 2002.

8. LeVoyer T, Cioffi WG Jr, Pratt L, Shippee R, McManus WF, Mason AD Jr, Pruitt BA, Jr. Alterations in intestinal permeability after thermal injury. Arch Surg 127(1):26-29, 1992.

9. Sefton EJ, Boulton-Jones JR, Anderton D, Teahon K, Knights DT. Enteral feeding in patients with major burn injury: The use of nasojejunal feeding after the failure of nasogastric feeding. Burns 28(4):386-390, 2002.

10. Sheridan RL, Weber JM, Pasternack MS, Tompkins RG. Antibiotic prophylaxis for group A streptococcal burn wound infection is not necessary. J Trauma 51(2):352-355, 2001.

11. Thompson JT, Meredith JW, Molnar JA. The effect of burn nursing units on burn wound infections. J Burn Care Rehabil 23(4):281-286, 2002.

12. Williams RM, Patterson DR, Schwenn C, Day J, Bartman M, Engrav LH. Evaluation of a peer consultation program for burn inpatients. 2000 ABA paper. J Burn Care Rehabil 23(6):449-453, 2002.

13. Artz CP, Gibson T. Management of burns. Mil Med 141(10):673-679, 1976.

14. Demling RH. Medical progress: Burns. N Engl J Med 313(22)1389-1398, 1985.

15. Ripbson MC, Burns BF, Smith DJ Jr. Acute management of the burned patient. Plast Reconstr Surg 89(6):1155-1168, 1992.

16. Nguyen TT. Current treatment of severely burned patients. Ann Surg 223(1):14-25, 1996.

17. Kao CC, Garner WL. Acute burns. Plast Reconstr Surg 101(7):2482-2493, 2000.

18. Rosenkranz KM, Sheridan R. Management of the burned trauma patient: Balancing conflicting priorities. Burns 28(7):665-669, 2002.

4 ▪ Wound Care, Use of Antibiotics, and Control of Burn Wound Sepsis

The rate of survival in burn patients has improved considerably over the past few decades. This can be attributed to advances in resuscitation, nutritional support, pulmonary care, wound care, and infection control. Sepsis is the leading cause of death in patients with large burns[1]; 75% of all deaths following burn injury are related to infection. Ninety-one percent of patients dying with burn wound sepsis have positive bacterial or fungal cultures.[2]

In the 1940s early mortality of burn patients was usually caused by shock. After the Coconut Grove nightclub tragedy in Boston, in which 492 persons died, aggressive resuscitation with fluid and electrolytes became standard practice.[3] Patients typically would live an average of 3 days, only to die from *Streptococcus* sepsis. In 1945 the use of penicillin, along with fluid and electrolyte management, became the standard of treatment. Patients then typically died 2 weeks later from penicillin-resistant *Staphylococcus*. During the 1950s penicillin-resistant antibiotics were developed. Patients then succumbed to infection by gram negative organisms. Infection with *Pseudomonas* organisms began to be seen in increasing numbers.[4] The organisms faced by patients range from the common nosocomial bacteria (e.g., *Staphylococcus* and beta-hemolytic *Streptococcus*, *Pseudomonas aeruginosa*, and *Escherichia coli*) to more exotic bacteria selected out by widespread antibiotic use, such as methicillin-resistant *Staphylococcus aureus* (MRSA), *Klebsiella*, *Enterobacter*, *Proteus*, *Provodentia*, and *Serratia*.[5]

Individual hospital units will notice a change in their common pathogens over time, and continued surveillance is essential. Fungal infection with such organisms as *Candida albicans* is on the increase. Prevention continues to be a cornerstone of infection control.[6]

PATHOPHYSIOLOGY

With a burn injury, the normal skin barrier against bacteria is lost. This is also combined with local release of cytokines, immune-suppressive factors, ischemia (with breakdown of normal tissue and circulating cellular components), wound maceration, high moisture content, and acidic pH. Later, endotoxins, exotoxins, and enzymes from microbes have local and systemic effects. This subsequently leads to hypermetabolism and catabolism, eventually depleting energy stores and decreasing the body's resistance to infection.[7,8] Blood supply to the wound is usually compromised, secondary to edema and thrombosis of the vasculature by the thermal injury.

Microbes may descend through the eschar and enter the sub-eschar plane. Enzymes released by microorganisms and WBCs cause lysis of denatured burn wound proteins. This provides more nutritional substrates for the bacteria. Bacterial growth can sometimes be held in check at the interface between the eschar and the viable tissue. Topical administration of antibiotics is helpful to distribute the antimicrobial compound at the involved site.[6] Topical agents will not sterilize a burn wound. Their use is intended to control bacterial growth on the burn wound.[9-11]

Further breakdown of host defenses may tip the balance in favor of the bacteria advancing into the adjacent healthy tissue. Hematogenous spread follows invasion of bacteria into the viable tissues.

The goals of treatment for a burn patient include the prevention of sepsis, as well as the preservation of function and form.

The management of burn wounds is part of the overall treatment strategy. This includes many aspects of the patient's care. Resuscitation is important to ensure adequate cardiopulmonary function—

essential for tissue perfusion as well as immunologic reserve for wound healing and prevention of burn sepsis. Cardiopulmonary function is also significant for nutrition, antibiotics, and oxygen transport to the tissues. If there is no cardiopulmonary function, the necessary materials needed cannot travel from where they are to where they are needed (e.g., intravenous antibiotics need to travel through the bloodstream to the infected area).

Advances in critical care have also contributed to the improvement in the management of the burn patient. The ability to monitor perfusion and fluid status in the resuscitative period and beyond has greatly improved. One can see early changes in cardiac function, systemic perfusion, or sepsis.

Improvements in the understanding and management of the nutritional needs of this unique population have improved outcomes. The burn patient has very high metabolic needs, with an increase in the basic metabolic rate as high as 2 to 2.5 times the basic energy expenditure. The role of early enteric support has also been appreciated. This is seen in the preservation of the integrity of the bowel lumen and subsequent prevention of translocation of bacteria and cytokines across the bowel wall. This may decrease susceptibility to infection.[12] The support of immune system is also important as profound immunosuppression usually follows major injury.[2,13]

Decreasing bacterial translocation of bacteria, cytokines, and endotoxins may help decrease the manifestations of systemic infection. The intent is not to sterilize the bowel per se, but to decrease the amount of bacteria and toxins that may travel across the bowel wall. Support of the mucosa is important, as mentioned earlier. Indications for this therapy are burns greater than 20% TBSA.

Control of translocation may afford an additional local benefit in the pulmonary tissue (in light of the lymphatic flow drawing from the peritoneal cavity toward the diaphragm), where translocated bacteria and toxins may compound the insults of smoke inhalation and respiratory depression that can contribute to increased rates of pulmonary infection. Pneumonia is a well-known and significant complication in this patient population.

The isolation of burn patients is associated with decreased incidence of gram negative sepsis and improved survival.[14]

COMMON PATHOGENS

There are certain bacteria typically found in burn wounds. Principally gram positive bacteria isolated from burn wounds are staphylococci and beta-hemolytic streptococci. The most common gram-negative bacteria are *P. aeruginosa* and *E. coli*. Other gram negative organisms seen include *Klebsiella, Enterobacter, Proteus, Provodentia*, and *Serratia*. Fungi, especially *Candida albicans*, are also seen.[5]

The most common causative organisms of burn sepsis are gram negative bacilli. These include *E. coli, Klebsiella, Enterobacter, Proteus, Provideiicia, Serratia marcescens*, and *P. aeruginosa*. These frequently found to be nosocomial organisms that may be resistant to conventional antibiotic therapy. *Staphylococcus aureus* is also a significant cause of infection in burn patients. Methicillin-resistant *S. aureus* (MRSA) may also arise in some burn units.[5]

INITIAL MANAGEMENT OF THE WOUND

Louis Pasteur stated, "The germ is nothing, it is the terrain in which it grows which is everything."[15] The eschar is known to be an excellent culture medium. This avascular space will eventually become colonized with bacteria. In fact, it may become colonized despite application of topical antibiotics. Our institution uses a collagenase/polysporin powder. This provides antibiotic protection and will help loosen the eschar for eventual debridement.

The cornerstone of burn wound care is the prompt excision of necrotic tissue and closure of the wound with skin grafts or biologic dressings. Host resistance can now be adequately protected and the possibility of wound contamination minimized.[6] Early wound closure may be associated with lower rates of infection and mortality.[16] Our institution will perform an escharectomy for full-thickness burns on days 3 to 5. Escharotomy for partial-thickness burns are performed on or about day 18. These guidelines also take into consideration clinical evaluation, coloration, and consistency of the wound and patient's condition. Excised eschar is sent for culture and sensitivities. A wound biopsy is performed in the first week. Biopsies are not typically performed after 2 weeks.

In patients with large areas of unequivocal full-thickness burns, direct excision to fascia is the procedure of choice. In patients with mixed deep dermal and full-thickness injuries, or in those in whom the exact area of full-thickness burn is difficult to determine, sequential eschar excisions are performed.

Larger burns may require staged excision and often allograft closure. Fresh donor sites are also at risk for infection. Superficial second-degree burns that are not excised also need protection.

A variety of modalities can now be used to cover the burn. As stated previously, early excision and coverage affords the patient less risk of infection, decreased metabolic work, and subsequent better outcome.

Split-thickness skin grafts can be used to cover partial-thickness burns. Such grafts use the patient's own tissue and are a mainstay of treatment. One disadvantage is that the donor site is now also a wound that needs to heal. If a patient has massive wounds, harvesting additional skin may not be an option. The patient may have "run out of skin" (e.g., a patient with a 60% burn leaves only 40% skin left). One clearly cannot use all of the remaining skin (e.g., harvesting from the face), so the patient needs an alternative form of coverage for the debrided wound.

Temporary coverage is often a viable alternative. Cadaver skin and pigskin can be used in this manner. Such a graft will eventually slough off, but it will buy time until the body is less hypermetabolic and more of the patient's own skin can be used.

Permanent coverage using various commercial modalities is now possible. Alloderm is a cultured, processed dermis that aids in graft take and serves as a biologic scaffold for normal tissue remodeling. The meshed Alloderm is placed on the burn wound, and a skin graft is placed on top of the Alloderm. Histologically, one cannot tell from the dermis that the patient has been burned. However, the difference is there are no sweat glands or hair follicles seen. We use this modality in large burn wounds.

Integra is another modality currently in use. This product, billed as "skin off the shelf," is made from bovine connective tissue. Strips of Integra are placed on the wound as a skin graft would be. We have used this modality on significant size wounds to achieve coverage in one sitting. This modality has been especially effective on wounds across joints, with improved range of motion.

Although most grafts take in the first few days after a burn injury, seldom is complete closure accomplished. Protection from infection is still required.

Protection from infection includes recognizing personnel and family as potential sources of contamination. Isolation measures are necessary, such as gowning of caregivers and use of patient-specific items. The importance of hand-washing must be stressed.

INFECTED WOUNDS

Infected wounds are a serious problem in burn patients. Infection does not allow the burn to heal. Infection delays epidermal maturation and leads to additional scar tissue formation.[17] Infection continues to stimulate the patient's hypermetabolic state. Treatment includes clysis, as guided by biopsy. Clysis is a procedure in which a substance—in this case, antibiotics—are injected under the plane of tissue. Clysis can be used to separate the skin layer from the underlying tissue, and may also be done for control of operative blood loss. For example, one ampule of epinephrine can be mixed with 1 L of normal saline solution, then clysis is performed. Parenteral antibiotics are indicated when wound biopsies show bacteria counts of greater than 1×10^5 per cubic centimeter of tissue. This is also the point at which healing of the wound is compromised. Parenteral antibiotics are not usually given until just before surgery, or in the case of burn wound infection.[18-20]

PREOPERATIVE PARENTERAL ANTIBIOTICS

Preoperative parenteral antibiotics are selected against the organism found in the biopsy.[16] These are administered before the operation because of the bacteremia produced at time of operation.[21] Parenteral antibiotics should cover *P. aeruginosa* and staphylococci.[22] Choices of antibiotics include vancomycin and amikacin, nafcillin and an aminoglycoside, or antipseudomonal penicillin and aminoglycoside. Alternative treatments include a cephalosporin and an aminoglycoside, vancomycin and an aminoglycoside.[5] Amikacin is becoming a preferred substitution for aminoglycoside. Imipenem has been shown to be very useful, especially postoperatively, as guided by culture data.

TETANUS PROPHYLAXIS

A burn patient has an open wound. In our institution standard practice is to administer tetanus immune globulin prophylactically to patients who have not had such prophylaxis in the past 5 years.

TOPICAL ANTIBIOTICS

Topical antibiotics control microbiologic invasion of open wounds much more effectively than do systemic antibiotics.[9,10] The choice of a topical antibiotic should follow the general rules outlined above. They are intended to limit colonization and to control growth of pathologic organisms. Topical antibiotics may decrease cytokines and chemical mediators. They may act by changing the chemical makeup of the burn wound milieu rather than the actual bacteriostatic or bactericidal component of use. Some institutions change the topical antibiotics every 7 days to increase the effectiveness and decrease the possibility of selecting out resistant strains of pathogens. Use of the topical antibiotic is guided first empirically, or by the resident flora of the individual burn unit. One should note whether the patient arrived after being in an institution (e.g., nosocomial infection in nursing home residents who sustain burn injury and are admitted to the burn unit).[23]

We recommend applying topical agent to the dressing and then applying it to the wound. This is more comfortable for the patient and prevents contamination of the topical agent's receptacle by contact with the patient's burned skin.

Collagenase/Polysporin Powder. Collagenase/polysporin powder has become the first-line choice in our institution. It is effective, well tolerated, and in keeping with the total management plan of the patient (i.e., removal of dead tissue/culture medium eschar). This modality also affords antimicrobial coverage.[11]

Silver Sulfadiazine (Silvadene). Silver sulfadiazine is the most commonly used topical antibiotic. It is used extensively for outpatient treatment as well as in the inpatient setting. It has excellent broad-spectrum coverage and is also effective against *Candida*. It may be used with or without a dressing. It is painless and easy to apply. Drawbacks include leukopenia and poor eschar penetration.

Our institution uses it as a first-line outpatient and inpatient topical antibiotic.

Betadine, a 10% Ointment of Povidone-Iodine. Povidone-iodine ointment has broad antimicrobial properties. Its main active ingredient is iodine. It can be used on open or closed wounds. The best antimicrobial activity is seen if it is administered every 6 hours. It can produce pain, immune depression, kidney dysfunction, and thyroid dysfunction. This modality should not be used in children and pregnant women because of the potential for iodine toxicity. The main use at this time is to prepare a wound for excision by making the surface hard, mechanically allowing easier incision.

Silver Nitrate, AgNO₃ 0.5% Solution. Silver nitrate is a broad-spectrum bacteriostatic topical agent that is painless to apply. It has limited eschar penetration (like Silvadene), because the silver is quickly bound to the body's natural chemical compounds, such as chloride. It is light sensitive, turning black on contact with tissues and chloride-containing substances. The agent leaches NaCl from the tissue, so hyponatremia may become a problem. Monitoring of electrolytes is important. The agent may also cause methemoglobinemia, because the organisms will break the compound down from NO_3 to NO_2 form, which is now absorbed by the patient. Bulky cotton dressings, thicker than 1 inch, are used. Soaks every 2 hours around the clock along with twice-daily dressing changes are needed. Hypothermia is also an issue with this treatment because of silver nitrate's evaporative cooling effect. Remember that the burn patient must be kept warm. This agent is used only in specialized units.

Mafanide Acetate (Sulfamyelon). Mafanide acetate gives excellent penetration of full-thickness eschar. It is equal in efficacy to Silvadene against gram negative organisms. It decreases bacteria counts and is easy to apply. It is especially effective against *Clostridia* and *Pseudomonas* organisms. It has a narrow spectrum of activity, mostly against gram negative rods. It does not affect *Candida*. It can cause metabolic acidosis, because it is a carbonic anhydrase inhibitor. Rarely, it can cause an aplastic crisis. Caution is needed when using it on a greater than 70% TBSA wound, because of the potential for a metabolic acidosis. This modality may cause pain to the patient when applied.

Gentamicin. Gentamicin is an antibiotic that decreases wound colonization against *Pseudomonas*. Rapidly emerging resistant organisms sometimes prohibit its use. This drug is also not often used systemically because of the selection of resistant organisms in the wound. Amikacin is becoming a preferred substitution for the aminoglycosides.

Nystatin, Myconizole to Control *Candida, Phycomycetes*. These antifungal agents are mixed with mafinide or sulfadiazine and applied topically to control *Candida*. Nystatin oral wash (swish) is used to control thrush, especially with concomitant antibacterial usage. This may assume more of a role in the future, because the use of wide-spectrum antibiotics is changing the flora found in burn units and burn wounds.

SYSTEMIC ANTIFUNGAL AGENTS

Amphotericin B. Amphotericin B has long been used as a systemic antifungal agent. Dosing includes setting a goal dose (6 mg/kg), then working up to it. The usual starting dose is 0.25 to 0.50 mg/kg. The duration of therapy then depends on how long it takes to reach the goal dose. One should apply a test dose (1 mg in 100 ml) before starting therapy. The normal concentration of amphotericin B is 0.1 mg/ml. The drug has side effects that include fever, nausea, vomiting, and hypokalemia.

Diflucan. Fluconazole (Diflucan) is a newer systemic antifungal agent. It is effective and does not have the unique dosing necessary or the profound side effects of amphotericin. This agent may have an increasing role in the near future. It is our institution's first-line parenteral antifungal agent. Other systemic antifungal agents will soon be available and should help to address the increasing incidence of fungal infection.

UNIQUE POPULATION

Burn patients are unique in many ways. The metabolic stress, pathophysiology, and cutaneous wound of a burn injury all have systemic effects. The psychologic aspects of self-image as well as physiologic factors (e.g., range of motion, mobility) are distinct from those encountered in other patient populations.

Basic surgical principles are of paramount importance. Debridement of tissue, control of infection, nutritional and physiologic support, and prevention of sepsis all may be magnified in burn patients. The role of the burn surgeon is to attempt to control the many variables to achieve the best possible outcome.

Most wounds will become contaminated in a few days. There is therefore a "golden period" for excisional therapy of 5 to 7 days. After this time, patients undergoing excision will be subjected to bacteremia during excision of the eschar. Prophylactic antibiotics are given to cover this problem.

Antibiotic therapy, guided by clinical evaluation and cultures, must be tailored to the individual patient.[24]

REFERENCES

1. Edwards-Jones V, Greenwood JE. Manchester Burns Research Group. What's new in burn microbiology? James Laing Memorial Prize Essay 2000. Burns 29(1):15-24, 2003.
2. Hansbrough JF. Burn wound sepsis. J Intensive Care Med 2:313-327, 1987.
3. Saffle JR. The 1942 fire at Boston's Coconut Grove nightclub. Am J Surg 166(6):581-591, 1993.
4. Krizek T. Local factors influencing incidence of wound sepsis. Symposium on antibiotic prophylaxis and therapy. Contemp Surg 10:45-50, 1977.
5. Lampe KF. Antimicrobial therapy and chemoprophylaxis of infectious diseases. In Drug Evaluations, 6th ed. Chicago: American Medical Association, 1986, pp 1231-1232.
6. Mousa HA, al-Bader SM. Yeast infection of burns. Mycoses 44(5):147-149, 2001.
7. Pruitt BA Jr, McManus AT. Opportunistic infections in severely burned patients. Am J Med 76:146-154, 1984.
8. Pruitt BA Jr. Host-opportunistic interactions in surgical infection. Arch Surg 121:13-22, 1986.
9. Lampe KF. Topical anti infective agents: Drugs used on skin and mucous membranes. In Drug Evaluations, 6th ed. Chicago: American Medical Association, 1986, pp 1505-1507.
10. Moncrief JA. Topical antibacterial treatment of the burn patient. In Artz CP, Moncrief JA, Pruitt BA Jr, eds. Burns: A team approach. Philadelphia: WB Saunders, 1979, pp 250-299.
11. Hansbrough JF, Achauer B, Dawson J, Himel H, Luterman A, Slater H, Levenson S, Salzberg CA, Hansbrough WB, Dore C. Wound healing in partial thickness burns treated with collagenase ointment vs. silver sulfadiazine cream. J Burn Care Rehabil 16(3):241-247, 1995.

12. LeVoyer T, Cioffi WG Jr, Pratt L, Shippee R, McManus WF, Mason AD Jr, Pruitt BA Jr. Alterations in intestinal permeability after thermal injury. Arch Surg 127(1):26-29, 1992.

13. McCampbell B, Wasif N, Rabbitts A, Staiano-Coico L, Yurt RW, Schwartz S. Diabetes and burns: Retrospective cohort study. J Burn Care Rehabil 23(3):157-166, 2002.

14. McManus AT, Mason AD Jr, McManus WF, Pruitt BA Jr. A decade of reduced gram negative infections and mortality associated with improved isolation of burned patients. Arch Surg 129(12):1306-1309, 1994.

15. Pasteur L. Memoire sur les corpuscles organises qul existent, dans l'atmosphere: Examen de la doctrine des generations spontances, Annales Sciences Naturelles 16:5-98, 1861.

16. Sheridan RL, Weber JM, Pasternack MS, Tompkins RG. Antibiotic prophylaxis for group A streptococcal burn wound infection is not necessary. J Trauma 51(2):352-355, 2001.

17. Singer AJ, McClain SA. Persistent wound infection delays epidermal maturation and increases scarring in thermal burns. Wound Repair Regen 10(6): 372-377, 2002.

18. Keen A, Knoblock L, Edelman L, Saffle J. Effective limitation of blood culture use in the burn unit. J Burn Care Rehabil 23(3):183-189, 2002.

19. Santucci SG, Gobara S, Santos CR, Fontana C, Levin AS. Infections in a burn intensive care unit: Experience of seven years. J Hosp Infect 53(1):6-13, 2003.

20. Appelgren P, Bjornhagen V, Bragderyd K, Jonsson CE, Ransjo U. A prospective study of infections in burn patients. Burns 28(1):39-46, 2002.

21. Sasaki TM, Welch GW, Herndon DN, Kaplan JZ, Klindberg RB, Pruitt BA Jr. Burn wound manipulation induced bacteremia. J Trauma 19(1):46-48, 1979.

22. Estahbanati HK, Kashani PP, Ghanaatpisheh F. Frequency of *Pseudomonas aeruginosa* serotypes in burn wound infections and their resistance to antibiotics. Burns 28(4):340-348, 2002.

23. Signorini M, Grappolini S, Magliano E, Donati L. Updated evaluation of the activity of antibiotics in a burn centre. Burns 18(6):500-503, 1992.

24. Demling RH. Medical progress: Burns. N Engl J Med 313(22):1389-1398, 1985.

5 ▪ Nutrition

Nutrition is of crucial importance in the care of the burn patient. A burn patient is in a hypermetabolic state. This hypermetabolism is typically proportional to the extent of the injury and the accompanying responses, infections, and complications. A 50% increase in metabolism is expected in patients with multiple blunt injuries, central nervous system injuries, and major abdominal injuries, whereas a 100% increase in metabolism may be seen in patients with major burn injuries.[1]

It has been shown in burn patients that both the cardiac index and oxygen consumption are proportional to the severity of injury.[2] The upper limit of hypermetabolism seems to be 2 to 2.5 times the basal metabolic rate (BMR).[3] There is an increased rate of caloric expenditure and protein catabolism resulting from the increased levels of catecholamines, glucagon, and glucocorticoids.[4] Moderate to severe stress can cause nutritional depletion, depression of the immune system, decreased protein stores, diminished inflammatory response, and wound healing interference.[1]

INJURY, METABOLIC RATE, AND STRESS FACTORS

The relative effects of injury on metabolism can be seen below[5]:

Injury	Incidence in metabolic activity (%)	Stress factor
Elective operation	0-5	1.00-1.05
Long-bone fracture	15-30	1.15-1.30
Multiple trauma	30-55	1.30-1.55
Multiple trauma and sepsis	50-75	1.50-1.75
10% Burn	25	1.25
20% Burn	50	1.50
30% Burn	70	1.70
40% Burn	85	1.85
50% Burn	100	2.00
75% Burn	100-110	2.00-2.10

A burn patient loses large amounts of heat through wounds, as previously discussed. This may be another contributing factor in the hypermetabolism that occurs. Interestingly, in one study, burn patients' core and skin temperatures and metabolic rate continued to be elevated, even when the net heat loss was reduced by using increasing ambient temperatures.[6] When the burn patients were allowed to select their most comfortable ambient temperature, they consistently chose warmer temperatures than the control group did. The findings were explained as a response to the injury increasing the central temperature set-point of the patient.[3]

The body's response to stress includes protein catabolism, with subsequent urinary nitrogen loss and muscle wasting. Each gram of nitrogen represents 6.25 g of protein (roughly 20 g of muscle). A patient undergoing starvation (e.g., an NPO patient) loses about 75 g of muscle protein per day (roughly 200 to 300 g of muscle tissue). A 60% increase in metabolism can translate into a loss of 250 g of muscle protein per day (roughly 750 to 1000 g of muscle mass). The protein is broken down via deamination of amino acids to provide carbon skeletons for glucose production (e.g., gluconeogenesis in the liver). This breakdown is, again, proportional to the severity of stress.[7]

Skeletal muscle is the largest source of protein stores. These protein stores are utilized after burn injury. Indeed, in a study in which amino acid release from the legs of patients with major burns was measured, a fivefold increase was noted in the release of amino acid nitrogen.[8] Branched-chain amino acids (BCAAs) are leucine, isoleucine, and valine. They are oxidized primarily in muscle, and breakdown of muscle releases these amino acids in large amounts. They are also known to stimulate the secretion of insulin.[9] Providing high levels of BCAAs in nutritional support may decrease muscle breakdown; however, more studies are needed before a definitive statement can be made.[1]

Glutamine is a unique amino acid; it is sometimes referred to as a *conditionally essential* amino acid. The requirements of glutamine may be significantly increased in a stressed patient. Glutamine represents one third of nitrogen derived through catabolic metabolism of amino acids.[9] Glutamine is used for a wide variety of purposes.[9] This is especially true for the rapidly dividing cells of the GI tract. Glutamine-enriched parenteral nutrition nourishes the enterocytes, protects against atrophy of the intestinal mucosa, and improves nitrogen retention.[10] Maintenance of intestinal integrity may decrease translocation of bacteria and cytokines across the GI barrier, thus decreasing the incidence of sepsis.[11-13] Provision of glutamine may also be important for maintenance of the patient's immunologic responses.[14] Levels of glutamine are decreased in stress states, and glutamine needs to be a part of the nutritional plan.[9,15]

Hyperglycemia is noted after injury and is primarily caused by increased glucose production. The extra glucose comes from synthesis from amino acids and glucose recycled from lactate. Elevations of the fasting glucose and serum insulin concentrations occur. The elevations are not proportionate, and there may be a disturbance of the normal insulin-glucose relationship and insulin resistance.[3,16]

Lipolysis is also increased by several mechanisms—the firing of sympathetic nerves liberates adipose stores as well as increased levels of cortisol, catecholamines, and glucagon. This lipolysis is not suppressed by increased glucose levels. However, the availability of lipid is decreased as the circulation to the adipose tissue is impaired, decreasing free fatty acid (FFA) mobilization. The body may not be able to utilize triglycerides and FFA, because the activity of lipoprotein lipase may decrease.[17] Hormone-sensitive lipase (the lipase found in cells that actively breaks down triglycerides in adipose sites) may also be decreased.

These metabolic findings are coordinated to elicit a response beneficial to the patient. Multiple organ systems work together to attempt to supply injured tissue with the oxygen and metabolites needed for healing. They are regulated by neuroendocrine pathways via a variety of agents (cortisol, glucagon, thyroid hormones, catecholamines, insulin, growth hormone, and cytokines).[16,18]

NUTRITIONAL SUPPORT FOR THE INJURED PATIENT

Early and adequate nutritional support will minimize lean body mass catabolism, improve immune function, and protect protein synthesis. Enteral feedings are safer and less expensive than parenteral feedings and should be used whenever possible. Enteral feedings also protect the integrity of the bowel lumen[17]; this will decrease bacterial and toxin translocation into the peritoneal space and bloodstream.[11] Limiting translocation will decrease cytokine responses and involvement of the lungs (as the peritoneal lymph channels move lymph toward the diaphragm). In our institution, enteral feedings are started as soon as feasible. When the patient is admitted the stomach is emptied by an NGT, and 100 ml of a high glutamine feeding formula is administered in the stomach. The tube is clamped for 30 to 45 minutes. The NGT is then placed to suction and enteral feedings are begun if the gastric residuals are less than 100 ml/hr and active bowel sounds are present. An enteral tube with two ports is placed, one port to feed distal to the pylorus and the other port to decompress the stomach.[19]

Caloric and Protein Needs

Determining the patient's energy needs and BMR is necessary for the initiation of nutritional support. This is an estimate, a starting point. Adjustments will be made after evaluation of nutritional parameters. There are many formulas one can use to estimate the basal energy expenditure (BEE).

- A common and accurate formula is the Harris-Benedict equation[20]:

Basal Energy Expenditure (BEE)
Male =
66.5 + (13.7 × Weight in kg) + (5 × Height in cm) − (6.8 × Age)
Female =
65.5 + (9.6 × Weight in kg) + (1.7 × Height in cm) − (4.7 × Age)

Use the patient's normal weight for the calculation. Patients will gain a significant amount of weight with edema from the fluid resuscitation.

A stress factor needs to be added to the BEE to account for the increased metabolic needs of the patient. Burns greater than 20% of body surface area cause severe stress, and the BMR should be multiplied by a factor of 2. Burns less than 20% have a moderate stress level, and the BMR should be multiplied by a factor of 1.6.

- There is an alternative method to obtain a starting point. The caloric requirement can be estimated at 40 to 50 Kcal/kg for severe stress. For moderate stress, the estimated need is 35 to 40 Kcal/kg.

- Another method: Estimate the basal energy expenditure at 25 Kcal/kg, then multiply it by the aforementioned stress factor (i.e., 1.6 for moderate stress, 2.0 for high stress).

- Yet another method is the Curreri formula:

Amount of calories needed =
$$(25 \text{ Kcal} \times \text{kg}) + (40 \text{ Kcal} \times \% \text{TBSA})$$

There are a variety of other ways to accurately calculate the energy expenditure (e.g., the Fick principle and Weir equation, the metabolic cart, differential oximetry), but in clinical application, only a starting point is needed. The patient's nutritional status is monitored on a weekly basis (using prealbumin and transferrin levels). Some institutions now have hand-held metabolic cart units. The data at your institution can be evaluated and adjustments made.[21-23]

Fat is a dense source of calories. Usually, it is desirable for 30% of calories to come from fat. Special considerations in pulmonary disease may require an increase of fats up to 60% of the daily requirement to lower the respiratory quotient (CO_2/O_2) and decrease CO_2 production. In patients with respiratory difficulty, it may be advisable to give more calories as fat, so as to decrease the amount of CO_2 produced. This may improve the patient's respiratory status, and the patient may have an easier time weaning from the ventilator. The patient should receive at least 1000 Kcal/wk as fat so as to avoid essential fatty acid (EFA) deficiency.

Respiratory Quotient
>| Carbohydrates | 1.0 |
>|---|---|
>| Protein | 0.8 |
>| Lipids | 0.7 |

The normal respiratory quotient (RQ) is 0.8 in the average adult diet, consisting of 70% carbohydrate calories and 30% fat calories.

After estimating the caloric needs, one can calculate the protein needs. Protein calories "do not count" toward the caloric needs of the patient. Normal protein intake is 1 g/kg/day. Moderately stressed patients need 1.5 to 2.2 g of protein/kg/day. Patients with severe stress, such as a burn injury, require 2.2 to 3.2 g of protein/kg/day.

The ratio of calories to grams of nitrogen in a healthy, non-stressed individual is 300:1. In the hospital the ratio usually used is 150:1 (because the patients are usually under stress). The quotient is then multiplied by 6.25 (6.25 g of protein per gram of nitrogen). This gives the grams of protein needed. You'll note that the more stressed the patient is, the lower the calorie/nitrogen ratio (i.e., 100:1 for very stressed patients).

$$\frac{\text{Calories}}{150} \times 6.25 = \text{Grams of protein needed (for moderate stress)}$$

Protein Needs Vary With Stress
>| No stress | 1 g/kg/day |
>|---|---|
>| Moderate stress | 1.5-2.2 g/kg/day |
>| High stress | 2.2-3.2 g/kg/day |

Assessment of Protein Nutritional Status. The nitrogen balance (how much protein the patient needs) can be obtained from a 24-hour urinary urea nitrogen (UUN) measurement. The usual formula is:

Total nitrogen loss (TNL) = UUN + 4 g

6.25 g of protein are required to receive 1 g of biologically available nitrogen

Therefore

Protein needs = TNL × 6.25

The goal of therapy is a positive nitrogen balance of 2 to 4 g of nitrogen (15 to 30 g of protein) per day.[21] For example:

Protein Intake

$$\frac{\text{How many grams of protein you are giving}}{6.25} = \text{Grams of nitrogen you are giving}$$

Grams of nitrogen given − (UUN + 4) = Nitrogen balance (+ or −)

Again, you want the number to be positive.

Specifically in a burn patient, the TNL can be estimated as follows:

TNL = 2 + 24 hr UUN + Wound nitrogen loss

% Total burned surface area	Nitrogen/kg/day wound loss
<10%	0.02 g nitrogen/kg/day wound loss
11%-30%	0.05 g nitrogen/kg/day wound loss
>30%	1.2 g nitrogen/kg/day wound loss

This is an estimate of the initial needs of the patient. The patient requires monitoring of his or her nutritional status (usually once a week), and adjustments can be made accordingly. The UUN is an accurate estimate of the total urinary nitrogen in the burn-injured patient.[24]

Fluids

Use the Parkland formula as a starting point for fluid resuscitation.

Initial fluid replacement with lactated Ringer's solution is computed for the 24 hours of treatment. The equation, as mentioned before, is:

4 ml LR × Body weight in kg × %TBSA burn injury

Begin calculation of fluid resuscitation from the time of injury, not when the patient arrives at the ER. The first half of this volume is administered within 8 hours of the burn (even if there is a delay getting the patient to a medical center). The second half is given over the next 16 hours.

During the fourth 8-hour postburn period, salt-poor albumin (SPA) is infused using the equation (0.1 × kg × %TBSA). Water of evaporation must be calculated for burns greater than 25% TBSA and replaced as free water. This is so the patient does not become volume depleted.

The equation is:

%TBSA + (25 × BSA in m²) =
$\qquad$ Number of milliliters of evaporative water loss/hr

After the first 24-hour resuscitation period, maintenance fluid is D₅⅓NS. Maintenance fluids are based on the individual patient (see BSA calculation, p. 28), with close monitoring of his or her I&O. The rate is calculated for 24 hours by using this guideline:

First 10 kg	100 ml/kg
Second 10 kg	50 ml/kg
Every kg above 20 kg	20 ml/kg

For example, a 70-kg patient's calculation would be 100 × 10 (for the first 10 kg) + 50 × 10 (for the second 10 kg) + 50 × 20 (for the 50 other kg not covered yet): 1000 + 500 + 1000 = 2500 ml/24 hr. This totals 104 ml/hr. Remember, this is an estimate, and you can round up to more workable numbers (i.e., 105 ml/hr).

Electrolytes

The amount of sodium required ranges from 60 to 200 mEq/day. Less is required in patients with cardiac and renal failure. The amount of potassium needed is 50 to 160 mEq/day. Those patients who are stressed, on NGT suction, with a hyperinsulin state, or have a metabolic alkalosis require more. Chloride requirements are 100 to 200 mEq/day, more with gastric loss. Calcium requirements range from 4 to 30 mEq. Magnesium requirements are 8 to 24 mEq. Phosphate requirements are 30 to 100 mEq. In the burn unit the standard solution is $D_5\frac{1}{3}NS$ + 20 mEq KCl. This can be adjusted, and repletion of electrolytes can be given as guided by laboratory analysis.

Vitamins

Patients should receive a multivitamin and minerals, as seen in the initial orders section. Repletion of other vitamins and minerals may also be clinically based.[25]

Trace Elements

Trace elements are essential enzymatic cofactors in a variety of metabolic reactions. Zinc, manganese, copper, and chromium are added to parenteral solutions daily, along with the vitamins.

Zinc and iron levels are decreased by acute-phase reactants. The benefits of adding zinc are currently under much study. Bacteremia also tends to decrease the iron level. It is proposed that the bacteria need this element for biochemical reactions. There are ongoing studies evaluating withholding iron in septic patients. A study of patients with significant burns noted a decrease in the duration of hospitalization in the increased trace mineral intake group.[26]

Antioxidants

Antioxidants may prevent the damage caused by free radicals produced in the stress states. Copper and selenium are known to be involved in immune responses, oxidative defense mechanisms, and tissue repair[27]:

Nutrient	Activity
Vitamin C	Direct cytosolic antioxidant
Vitamin E	Direct antioxidant with action primarily at the cell membrane
Beta-carotene	Antioxidant properties, particularly at the membrane lipid
Zinc	Constituent of superoxide dismutase in cytosol
Manganese	Constituent of superoxide dismutase in mitochondria
Copper	Constituent of superoxide dismutase, and of the scavenger ceruloplasmin
Iron	Constituent of catalase
Selenium	Constituent of glutathione peroxidase
Glutamine	Substrate for endogenous glutathione

ENTERAL VERSUS PARENTERAL FEEDINGS

Most will agree that if the patient's gastrointestinal tract can be used, then it should be used. This will help maintain the benefits of nutritional support, including maintenance of the integrity of the gut (thus avoiding bacterial translocation). It will also avoid the possible complications of TPN. If the patient's GI tract cannot be accessed (guideline of 7 days), or if there is a contraindication to the enteral route, then nutritional support with a parenteral route is warranted.[19,28-30]

Complications of Parenteral Feedings	
Mechanical	Air or catheter embolism, pneumothorax, hemothorax, hydrothorax, arterial laceration, catheter-tip malposition, venous thrombosis
Infectious	Catheter-related sepsis

| Acute metabolic | Hyperglycemia, hypoglycemia, serum electrolyte abnormalities, fluid overload, hyperlipidemia |
| Prolonged use | Metabolic bone disease, intestinal mucosal atrophy, bacterial overgrowth, bacterial translocation, deterioration of liver function, alteration in bile composition |

There are many commercially available enteral feeding formulas. Dietitians can be quite valuable in selecting the proper formulation for the individual patient. In our burn unit, feedings are started immediately if possible. Determine the patient's BEE + stress factor. Now calculate the goal feeding that you want to achieve. The strength and rate of the feedings are increased per the protocol described next (if tolerated by the individual patient).

EXAMPLE: NPO if burn >30%:
    Enteral feedings, TraumaCal or similar
        Target feedings of 25 Kcal/kg/day × 2.0 (stress factor)
    Tube feedings:
        ½ strength @ 25 ml/hr × 4 hr, then
        ¾ strength @ 25 ml/hr × 4 hr, then
        Full strength @ 25 ml/hr × 4 hr, then
        Increase 15 ml/q4h to goal
    Check residuals q4h. Hold if <150 ml. If <150 ml, feed the aspirate back to the patient.

See Table 5-1 for a listing of the enteral feedings available. Note the location of the feeding catheter. In feedings to the stomach, one may increase tonacity first, followed by increased volume. Feedings to the small bowel are increased volume first, then tonicity (to avoid diarrhea). Remember to continue to assess the patient's nutritional status. Use the UUN to compute nitrogen balance and guide protein administration. Use transferrin, prealbumin, albumin to evaluate general nutritional therapy.

Table 5-1. Enteral feeding formulas

		Standard formulas		Specialty formulas: Disease specific				
	Product	Jevity	TwoCal HN	Nepro	Suplena	Pulmocare	NutriHep	Glucerna
1	Classification	Standard isotonic with fiber	2 Kcal/ml High calorie High protein	High calorie High protein Low electrolytes	High calorie Low protein Low electrolytes	Low carbohydrate	High branch chain amino acids (AA) Low aromatic AA	High fat Low CHO
2	Tube, oral, or both	Both	Both	Both	Both	Both	Both	Both
3	Calories/ml	1.06	2.0	2.0	2.0	1.5	1.5	1.0
4	Osmolality	310	690	635	600	475	690	355
5	Protein (g/ml)	0.044	0.084	0.070	0.030	0.063	0.040	0.042
6	Fat (g/ml)	0.035	0.091	0.096	0.095	0.093	0.021	0.054
7	Carbohydrate (g/ml)	0.152	0.217	0.215	0.255	0.106	0.290	0.096
8	Nonprotein Cal:N ratio	125:1	125:1	179:1	393:1	125:1	209:1	125:1
9	Protein source	Sodium & calcium caseinates	Sodium & calcium caseinates	Calcium, sodium, & magnesium caseinates	Sodium & calcium caseinates	Sodium & calcium caseinates	L-Amino acids Whey protein (50% BCAA)	Sodium & calcium caseinates
10	Fat source	High-oleic safflower oil (50%) Canola oil (30%) MCT oil (20%)	Corn oil MCT oil	High-oleic safflower oil (90%) Soy oil (10%)	High-oleic safflower oil (90%) Soy oil (10%)	Canola oil MCT oil Corn oil High-oleic safflower oil	MCT oil (66%) Canola oil Corn oil	High-oleic safflower oil Canola oil Soy lecithin
11	Carbohydrate source	Hydrolyzed cornstarch, soy polysaccharide	Maltodextrin, sucrose	Hydrolyzed cornstarch	Hydrolyzed cornstarch, sucrose, oat fiber, soy fiber	Sucrose, maltodextrin	Maltodextrin, modified cornstarch	Maltodextrin, soy fiber, fructose
12	Sodium (mg/ml)	0.930	1.456	0.829	0.783	1.310	0.320	0.930
13	Potassium (mg/ml)	1.570	2.456	1.057	1.116	1.730	1.360	1.570
14	Magnesium (mg/ml)	0.304	0.421	0.211	0.211	0.423	0.178	0.282
15	Phosphorus (mg/ml)	0.758	1.052	0.686	0.728	1.056	0.445	0.704
16	Calcium (mg/ml)	0.904	1.052	1.373	1.385	1.056	0.445	0.704
17	% Free water	84%	71%	70%	71%	79%	76%	87%
18	Milliliters needed to meet RDAs	1321	947	960 ml needed to meet RDAs, except Phos, Mg, vitamins A & D, which are limited in renal diets	947	947	1000	1422
19	Comments	Lactose free 14.4 g fiber/L	Concentrated for fluid restricted patients Lactose free Gluten free	Tailored for patients with renal failure who receive dialysis	Tailored for patients with renal failure, predialysis Gluten free Lactose free Low residue	Low CHO to reduce CO_2 production in respiratory failure Lactose free Gluten free	Tailored for chronic liver disease BCAA aromatic & methionine	Tailored for unstable diabetics whose blood sugars are out of control Not recommended for long-term use
20	Expense	$	$	$$	$	$	$$$$	$$
21	Supplier	Ross	Ross	Ross	Ross	Ross	Nestle	Ross

	Critical care formulas			Oral supplements per serving size					Tube feeding/Oral modifiers	
	Peptamen	Perative	Crucial	Ensure Plus	Resource	Ensure pudding	Health shakes	Sugar free health shakes	MCT oil	ProMod
1	Semi-elemental Isotonic	Semi-elemental High protein	Semi-elemental High protein	8 oz	8 oz clear liquid	5 oz	6 oz	6 oz	15 ml/Tbsp	6.6 g protein/scoop
2	Tube	Tube	Tube	Oral	Oral	Oral	Oral	Oral	Both	Both
3	1.0	1.3	1.5	355	180/8 oz	250/5 oz	280/6 oz	290/6 oz	7.75/ml	28 Kcal/scoop
4	270	385	490	450	700	—	—	—	—	5 g/scoop
5	0.04	0.067	0.094	13.2	8.8 g/8 oz	7 g/5 oz	9 g/6 oz	12 g/6 oz	14 g/Tbsp	—
6	0.039	0.038	0.068	12.7	0 g/8 oz	10 g/5 oz	6 g/6 oz	9 g/6 oz	—	—
7	127	0.177	0.135	48	36 g/8 oz	34 g/5 oz	48 g/6 oz	40 g/6 oz	—	—
8	131:1	97:1	67:1	150:1	105:1	230:1	—	—	—	—
9	Protein hydrolysate & peptides	Hydrolyzed sodium & caseinates & lactalbumin hydrolysates L-Arginine	Enzymatically hydrolyzed casein L-Arginine	Sodium & calcium caseinates soy protein isolate	Whey protein concentrate	Nonfat milk	Skim & nonfat dry milk	Skim milk, milk protein concentrate	—	Whey protein concentrate, soy lecithin
10	MCT oil (70%) Sunflower oil (30%)	Canola oil (40%) MCT oil (40%) Corn oil (20%)	MCT oil (50%) Marine oil (25%) Soy oil (25%)	Corn oil (100%)	No fat	Partially hydrogenated soybean oil	Corn oil	Corn oil	Medium chain triglycerides (100%)	—
11	Maltodextrin, cornstarch	Maltodextrin, cornstarch	Maltodextrin, cornstarch	Maltodextrin, sucrose	Sucrose, hydrolyzed cornstarch	Lactose, sucrose, modified food starch	—	—	—	—
12	0.500	1.040	1.170	280/8 oz	55/8 oz	239.2/5 oz	140/6 oz	240/6 oz	—	—
13	1.250	1.730	1.870	430/8 oz	15/8 oz	237/5 oz	400/6 oz	380/6 oz	—	—
14	0.400	0.347	0.400	100/8 oz	50/8 oz	68/5 oz	—	—	—	—
15	0.700	0.867	1.000	250/8 oz	160/8 oz	200/5 oz	—	—	—	—
16	0.800	0.867	1.000	250/8 oz	135/8 oz	200/5 oz	—	—	—	—
17	85%	79%	77%	182/8 oz	Approx 200 cc/8 oz	—	—	—	—	—
18	1500	1155	1000	1420	1900	Not applicable	—	—	—	—
19	For impaired GI function (i.e., short bowel syndrome, IBD, malabsorption, pancreatic insufficiency, chronic diarrhea, & radiation)	Lactose free L-Arginine & beta-carotene enriched	Lactose free Glutamine & arginine enriched	Lactose free Vanilla, chocolate, & strawberry	Clear liquid supplement Fat free Very low K+ & Na+ Low residue Lactose free	Gluten free Used for patients with impaired ability to swallow or fluid restriction NOT lactose free	House oral supplement	Diabetic house oral supplement	Supplemental MCT easily digested & absorbed	Supplemental high quality protein from whey Very low lactose
20	$$$$$	$$$	$$$$$	$	$	$	$	$	$$	$$
21	Nestle	Ross	Nestle	Ross	Sandoz	Ross	Sandoz	Sandoz	Ross	Ross

REFERENCES

1. Van Way CW III. Nutritional support in the injured patient. Surg Clin North Am 71(3):537-548, 1991.

2. Wilmore DW, Aulich LH, Mason AD, Pruitt BA Jr. Influence of the burn wound on local and systemic responses to injury. Ann Surg 186(4):444-458, 1977.

3. Bessey PQ. Parenteral nutrition and trauma. In Rombeau JL, Caldwell MD, eds. Clinical Nutrition: Parenteral Nutrition. Philadelphia: WB Saunders, 1993, pp 538-565.

4. Clifton GL, Robertson CS, Grossman RG, Hodge S, Foltz R, Garza C. The metabolic response to severe head injury. J Neurosurg 60(4):687-696, 1984.

5. Wilmore DW. The metabolic management of the critically ill. New York: Plenum, 1977, pp 149-152.

6. Wilmore DW, Mason AD Jr, Johnson DW, Pruitt BA Jr. Effect of ambient temperature on heat production and heat loss in burn patients. J Appl Physiol 38(4):593-597, 1975.

7. Goodwin C. Metabolism and nutrition in the thermally injured patient. Crit Care Clin 1(1):97-117, 1985.

8. Aulick LH, Wilmore DW. Increased peripheral amino acid release following burn injury. Surgery 85(5):560-565, 1979.

9. Wilmore DW. Catabolic illness. Strategies for enhancing recovery. N Engl J Med 325(10):695-702, 1991.

10. O'Dwyer ST, Smith RJ, Hwang TL, Wilmore DW. Maintenance of small bowel mucosa with glutamine-enriched parenteral nutrition. JPEN 13:579-585, 1989.

11. Maejima K, Deitch E, Berg RD. Bacterial translocation from the gastrointestinal tracts of rats receiving thermal injury. Infect Immun 43:86-102, 1984.

12. LeVoyer T, Cioffi WG Jr, Pratt L, Shippee R, McManus WF, Mason AD Jr, Pruitt BA Jr. Alterations in intestinal permeability after thermal injury. Arch Surg 127(1):26-29, 1992.

13. Wischmeyer PE, Lynch J, Liedel J, Wolfson R, Riehm J, Gottlieb L, Kahana M. Glutamine administration reduces gram-negative bacteremia in severely burned patients: A prospective, randomized, double-blind trial versus isonitrogenous control. Crit Care Med 29(11):2075-2080, 2001.

14. Lacey JM, Wilmore DW. Is glutamine a conditionally essential amino acid? Nutr Rev 48(8):297-309, 1990.

15. Souba WW, Klimberg VS, Plumley DA, Sallkoum RM, Flynn TC, Bland KI, Copeland EM III. The role of glutamine in maintaining a healthy gut and supporting the metabolic response to injury and infection. J Surg Res 48(4):383-391, 1990.

16. Thomas SJ, Morimoto K, Herndon DN, Ferrando AA, Wolfe RR, Klein GL, Wolf SE. The effect of prolonged euglycemic hyperinsulinemia on lean body mass after severe burn. Surgery 132(2):341-347, 2002.

17. Frankel WL, Evans NJ, Rombeau JL. Scientific rationale and clinical application of parenteral nutrition in critically ill patients. In Rombeau JL, Caldwell MD, eds. Clinical Nutrition: Parenteral Nutrition. Philadelphia: WB Saunders, 1993, pp 597-616.

18. Williams GJ, Herndon DN. Modulating the hypermetabolic response to burn injuries. J Wound Care 11(3):87-89, 2002.

19. McClave SA, Marsano LS, Lukan JK. Enteral access for nutritional support: Rationale for utilization. J Clin Gastroenterol 35(3):209-213, 2002.

20. Harris J, Benedict F. A biometric study of basal metabolism in man. Publ No. 279, Carnegie Institute of Washington. Philadelphia: JB Lippincott, 1919, as cited in American Dietetic Association Manual of Clinical Dietetics, Chicago, 1988.

21. Long CL, Schaffel N, Geiger JW, Schiller WR, Blacemore WS. Metabolic response to injury and illness: Estimation of energy and protein needs from indirect calorimetry and nitrogen balance. JPEN 3:452-457, 1979.

22. Williamson J. Actual burn nutrition care practices: A national survey (part II) J Burn Care Rehab 10(Pt 2):185-194, 1989.

23. Dickerson RN, Gervasio JM, Riley ML, Murrell JE, Hickerson WL, Kudsk KA, Brown RO. Accuracy of predictive methods to estimate resting energy expenditure of thermally-injured patients. JPEN 26(1):17-29, 2002.

24. Milner EA, Cioffi WG Jr, Mason AD Jr, McManus WF, Pruitt BA Jr. Accuracy of urinary urea nitrogen for predicting total urinary nitrogen in thermally injured patients. JPEN 17(5):414-426, 1993.

25. Van Way CW III. Vitamin and mineral deficiency. Handbook Surg Nutr 58:31-42, 1992.

26. Berger MM, Cavadini C, Chiolero R, Guinchard S, Krupp S, Dirren H. Influence of large intakes of trace elements on recovery after major burns. Nutrition 10(4):327-334, 1994.

27. Youn Y-K, LaLonde C, Demling R. Use of antioxidant therapy in shock and trauma. Circ Shock 35(4):245-249, 1991.

28. American Society for Parenteral and Enteral Nutrition (ASPEN). Guidelines for the use of parenteral and enteral nutrition in adult and pediatric patients. JPEN 17(4):1SA-52SA, 1993.

29. LeVoyer T, Cioffi WG Jr, Pratt L, Shippee R, McManus WF, Mason AD Jr, Pruitt BA Jr. Alterations in intestinal permeability after thermal injury. Arch Surg 127(1):26-29, 1992.

30. Kreis BE, Middelkoop E, Vloemans AF, Kreis RW. The use of a PEG tube in a burn centre. Burns 28(2):191-197, 2002.

6 ▪ Inhalation Injury

Inhalation injury is common, especially in patients with severe burn injuries. It is also an indicator of a poor prognosis. Mortality rates with inhalation injury usually are reported to be greater than 50%; this figure has changed little over the past 30 years. The incidence of inhalation injury is reported to be present in 3% to 21% of burn patients. The incidence rate is lower in children, in whom there is a higher percentage of scald injury than in adults. Inhalation injury can be diagnosed by history and physical examination, laboratory studies, chest radiographs, and fibroscopic examination. The pulmonary injury is usually proportional to the depth and size of the cutaneous burn.[1-3]

The injury can be acute, as seen in upper airway injury from heat damage, small airway damage from heat and particulate matter, and carbon monoxide poisoning. Toxins play a significant role, especially in victims of house fires, because many synthetic fabrics and home furnishings produce toxins when heated.[4]

Oxygen consumed during combustion decreases the ambient oxygen content in the air, exposing the person to a room with decreased oxygen content. This situation may lead to hypoxia in a person exposed to such an atmosphere for any length of time.

Carbon monoxide poisoning, which is also common in structural fires, can be diagnosed by unconsciousness, a change in mental status, and the results of laboratory studies (increased carboxyhemoglobin, low oxygen saturation in relation to PaO_2, and unexplained acidosis).

It can also result in the need for prolonged intubation. The classic cherry-red skin coloration associated with carbon monoxide poisoning is difficult to detect in burn patients. Symptoms will increase with increasing levels of carboxyhemoglobin level.[4-6]

Carboxyhemo- globin level	Symptoms
0-10	Normal
10-20	Slight headache, confusion, dilation of cutaneous blood vessels
20-30	Headache, throbbing in the temples
30-40	Disorientation, fatigue, nausea, vomiting, visual disturbances
40-60	Combativeness, hallucinations, shock state, coma, intermittent convulsions, Cheyne-Stokes respirations
>60	Mortality rate is >50%
60-70	Coma, intermittent convulsions, depressed cardiac and respiratory function
70-80	Weak pulse, slow respirations, death within hours
80-90	Death in less than 1 hour
90-100	Death within minutes

Treatment modalities include 100% oxygen administered by face mask. Treatment with 100% oxygen for 40 minutes will decrease the patient's carbon monoxide level by half.

Upper respiratory injury can be diagnosed by a history of fire in an enclosed space, burns of the face, singed nasal hair, inflamed pharyngeal mucosa, carbonaceous sputum, and evidence of edematous glottis (e.g., hoarseness). Any two of these clinical signs should prompt high suspicion of an inhalation injury. Worsening hoarseness, stridor, an increased respiratory rate, and inability to handle secretions demonstrate a worsening injury that will require intubation.

Bronchoscopy is warranted in patients with hoarseness or increasing hoarseness. Patients with stridor should be intubated *immediately*.

Signs of lower airway damage usually present within 24 hours after injury. Breath sounds characteristically are wheezing. Progressive hypoxemia may also be seen. Intubation should be considered after hypoxemia or edema is confirmed.

Oxygenation by intubation is a mainstay of treatment of a pulmonary injury. If the patient is awake and alert, nasotracheal intubation is preferred over orotracheal intubation and can be accomplished even if the patient's teeth are clenched. The oral route of intubation is less stable, but the danger of sinusitis is avoided. The endotracheal tube must be securely tied to ensure that the tube will not dislocate. Tape will not adhere to burned skin. Umbilical tape should be used and tied to the endotracheal tube and around the back of the head.

One of the new treatments for inhalation injury is inhaled nitrous oxide. This treatment is used to reduce a ventilation/perfusion (V/Q) mismatch by dilating the pulmonary vessels perfusing ventilated alveoli. Nitrous oxide inhalation therapy does not work well in bacteremic patients. Anecdotal success has been reported in the burn patient population.

Another new treatment modality is inhaled nebulized heparin mixed with albuterol. This has shown some success in decreasing airway casts.

A significant improvement has been the introduction of the Byrd ventilators. These combine oscillatory or high-frequency (500 to 800 beats/min) treatment with pressure-controlled breaths. The use of these ventilators has led to a decrease in inspiratory pressures and decreased barotraumas with sufficient oxygenation. The oscillatory breaths also provide internal chest physical therapy, mobilizing and decreasing particulate matter in the airway. Studies from the Institute of Surgical Research have shown decreased morbidity and mortality using this ventilator system.[7] In our burn unit use of these ventilators has also resulted in a decrease in the rate of pneumonia.

A circumferential chest burn may also cause respiratory embarrassment by restricting chest movement as a result of edema. The swelling is restricted by the eschar, which is nonelastic and therefore restricts chest excursion and breathing. An escharotomy may be necessary using the techniques previously described.

PATHOPHYSIOLOGY

Damage to the upper airway is manifested by edema, erythema, and ulceration. Edema results from direct microvascular injury, oxygen free radicals, and inflammatory mediators. Pulmonary edema formation usually begins immediately, or may be delayed up to 24 hours. Administration of crystalloid solution in and of itself does not seem to be a contributing factor in lung edema.[8] The tongue, arytenoids, and epiglottis may swell, narrowing or closing the airway. Because of the cartilaginous rings surrounding the glottis, swelling is displaced inward and narrows the airway. Edema usually resolves in 4 to 5 days. Decreases in upper airway edema can be estimated by evaluating the eyelids. When the edema of the eyelids has subsided, *in general,* the edema of the airway has also subsided and one may begin to consider extubation.[9,10]

In contrast to upper airway injury, the lower airways sustain less injury from dry heat. The upper airway can cool the warm air effectively. The vocal cords close at 302° F (150° C) and tend to serve as a protective measure. Steam has 4000 times the carrying capacity of dry air and can cause thermal injury. Smoke can also carry superheated particles or soot into the lower airway system. These particles cause direct thermal injury to the mucosa by contact. Small airway occlusion secondary to sloughed endobronchial debris and the loss of the ciliary clearance mechanism can result in a high rate of pneumonia (20% to 50%).[2] Various chemical agents (e.g., aldehydes, acroline, and acids) are released by burning. This is especially true of plastics, which can produce cyanide. Cyanide interferes with oxidative phosphorylation at the cellular level and causes a metabolic acidosis.

Specific treatment with sodium thiosulfate is not usually required in patients who have received adequate resuscitation and ventilation therapy.[11]

Constriction and obstruction of the airway cause vasoconstriction and hypoxia. Neutrophils are entrapped in the parenchyma, and the chemotactic factors released by those neutrophils recruit more neutrophils. Neutrophils release oxygen free radicals and proteolytic enzymes. Disruption of the interstitial matrix results in fluids and protein loss into the interstitial space.

TREATMENT

Treatment is designed to minimize the sequelae of pulmonary injury. One may consider free radical scavengers as well as the following.

Pulmonary Toilet

Chest physical therapy and postural drainage with frequent suctioning are required. Bronchoscopy is used to remove casts and debris, and brushings for culture are useful.[12]

Antibiotics

Prophylactic administration of antibiotics does not prevent bacterial pneumonia. Prophylactic antibiotics can select out resistant organisms; this may predispose the patient to worse pneumonia processes that are harder to eradicate. Appropriate antibiotics should be used for documented infections.

Steroids

Steroid medications reduce mucosal edema, blunt changes in capillary permeability, and stabilize cellular membranes and lysosomes. They may also inhibit the chemotactic action of the complement system. However, in burn patients the side effects of these drugs outweigh their theoretical benefits. Animal models have demonstrated increased mortality in steroid-treated groups, and an increased incidence of infection has been seen. These types of complications have also been documented in the adult burn population. In our unit and other units' experience, the use of steroids is not warranted in the treatment of burn patients.[11]

Ventilation/Oxygenation

Inverse-rate ventilation theoretically increases functional residual capacity. Mean pressures are increased without elevation of peak pressures. Pressure-control ventilation (PCV) delivers gas flow at a constant pressure. Tidal volume (VT) is determined by pressure. PCV lowers peak airway pressures and maintains minute ventilation. The pressure setting is obtained by dividing the tidal volume by the patient's compliance.

High-frequency ventilation (HFV) has been shown to be effective in several clinical trials in patients with isolated pulmonary injury. HFV is characterized by a ventilatory cycle greater than 60 breaths/min, lower peak airway pressures, and minimal FRC, and improved clearance of bronchial secretions.

Positive end-expiratory pressure (PEEP) improves oxygen saturation and reduces intrapulmonary shunting by recruiting alveoli. There is controversy that while receiving ventilatory therapy, patients should receive "physiologic levels" (i.e., 5 cm H_2O) of PEEP. PEEP has not been shown to improve overall outcomes, and has the potential to decrease cardiac output and cause barotrauma. However, one can increase oxygenation of the patient without increasing the FIO_2 to toxic levels. A "best PEEP" study can be done with the use of the SvO_2. One may dial in the PEEP using this number to titrate the amount. Wait 20 minutes after each change to ascertain the correct number. PEEP is also beneficial in patients with acute respiratory distress syndrome (ARDS) and postoperative atelectasis. The beneficial effects of PEEP are usually diminished over 15 cm H_2O.

Ventilator Management

It is essential to understand what the results of arterial blood gas (ABG) measurements mean and the appropriate responses in the acute, posttraumatic (burn), and/or postsurgical setting.[14]

ABG readings typically look like this: 7.40/40/90 (pH, P_{CO_2}, and P_{O_2}, respectively). This is all the information you need from the ABG slip to evaluate acute respiratory processes. The information received on the ABG can be broken down into two categories:

Oxygenation   or   Ventilation

Oxygenation is seen in the ABG as the P_{O_2}. There is a relationship between the P_{O_2} and the oxygen saturation. This is expressed as the oxygen-hemoglobin dissociation curve. Entities that move the curve to the right (offload oxygen into the bloodstream) include decreased pH, increased CO_2, increased temperature, and increased 2,3 DPG.

P_{O_2}	O_2 saturation
60	90
47	75
27	50

The normal relationship is reflected by these major points. Note that even at a P_{O_2} of 60, the saturation is still acceptable at 90%. After this point, there is a steep drop-off. Note also that you do not need the ABG to tell you the saturation—you already know it from the P_{O_2}. To emphasize: You need only three numbers from the ABG—pH, P_{CO_2}, and P_{O_2}.

Oxygenation is managed with the ventilator using FI_{O_2} and PEEP. One usually wishes to decrease the FI_{O_2} to under 60%, because oxygen levels this high are associated with toxicity to the lung tissues. There are exceptions, discussed earlier, in the burn population (e.g., carbon monoxide exposure). (See earlier PEEP discussion.)

Figure 6-1. Oxygen dissociation curve.
(Adapted from Simmons RL, Steed DL. Basic Science Review for Surgeons. Philadephia: WB Saunders, 1992.)

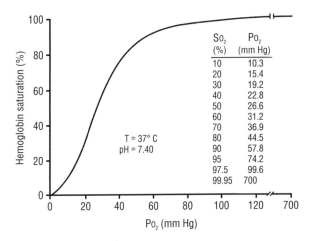

SO_2 (%)	PO_2 (mm Hg)
10	10.3
20	15.4
30	19.2
40	22.8
50	26.6
60	31.2
70	36.9
80	44.5
90	57.8
95	74.2
97.5	99.6
99.95	700

T = 37° C
pH = 7.40

Ventilation is managed using the minute ventilation:

Minute ventilation = Respiratory rate (RR) × Tidal volume (V_T)

One needs to determine whether there is an abnormality, diagnose the cause, and treat the problem. It is necessary to compute the *base deficit* or *excess* on each ABG. This is done the same way, each time. This way it becomes a habit, and the practitioner is less likely to "miss" abnormalities. A base deficit is also known as a *negative base excess*. Determine the base deficit yourself; your calculation is more accurate than the one on the ABG slip. Again, you only need three numbers on the ABG.

Determination of Base Deficit From ABG

1. A change in P_{CO_2} of 10 leads to a change in the pH (in the opposite direction).

   EXAMPLE
   a. If P_{CO_2} = 50, expect a decrease in the pH of 0.08. For simplicity, just say that the P_{CO_2} is "up" 10 and the pH is "down" 8.
   b. Discard the pH decimals, because they may confuse you.

2. Base deficit = ⅔ the difference between predicted pH (by P_{CO_2} alone) and the actual pH.

   EXAMPLE: pH 7.40, P_{CO_2} 30
   a. Based on the P_{CO_2} alone, the pH should be 7.48. The patient is "down" 10. So the patient's pH should be "up" 8 (7.40 + 0.08 = 7.48). But he is not.
   b. The measured pH from the ABG is 7.40. There is a difference between the predicted and the measured (7.40 − 7.48). This difference is 8 (again disregarding decimals).
   c. Take this number (8) and multiply it by ⅔ to get the base deficit or excess.

      8 × ⅔ = ¹⁶⁄₃, or approximately 5

   d. Now the pH is lower (more acidic) than expected, so there is a base deficit of 5 (or base excess of −5).
   e. The threshold for a diagnosis of a metabolic acidosis is usually a base deficit of 5. Acute metabolic acidosis is usually treated. The treatment is with HCO_3.

HCO_3 Replacement

1. The bicarbonate space (in liters) = (0.4) × (Body weight in kg) × (Base deficit).

   EXAMPLE: 0.4 × 70 kg × 5 = 140 mEq HCO_3

a. Replace HCO_3 by giving only half this amount (e.g., 70 mEq HCO_3).

b. One ampule of HCO_3 contains 50 mEq, so the dose is 1.5 ampules.

c. Whenever you make a ventilator change, give HCO_3, or provide any treatment that may affect the ventilation or acid/base status of a patient, check ABG 20 minutes after the intervention. Changes in oxygenation can be assessed with the pulse oximeter, although an occasional ABG measurement may be helpful.

d. Do not hesitate to increase minute ventilation to compensate for metabolic acidosis via generating a respiratory alkalosis.

e. Generally, base deficits of greater than 5 are treated with HCO_3 replacement.

f. Metabolic acidosis should be considered abnormal. Search for a reason why the patient is "making acid," and then treat the problem.

2. Respiratory acidosis or alkylosis may be managed by making changes on the ventilator settings. As described, one can help treat a metabolic acidosis by giving the patient a *small* respiratory alkalosis (on purpose).

Changing the Ventilator Setting to Change the CO_2

1. When adjusting the PCO_2, think as though the minute ventilation $(V_T \times RR)$ = Alveolar ventilation.

2. PCO_2 is inversely proportional to the minute ventilation (e.g., a larger minute volume will "blow off" PCO_2).

$$V_T \times Rate \times CO_2 \underset{Current}{} = V_T \times Rate \times CO_2 \underset{Desired}{}$$

EXAMPLE: A patient has a tidal volume of 1000 cc, a rate of 10, and a P_{CO_2} of 60. You want the P_{CO_2} to be 40.

a. Place the current numbers in the equation.

   $1000 \text{ V}_T \times \text{Rate } 10 \times 60 \text{ CO}_2$

b. Have the desired CO_2 equal what you want it to be.

   Desired CO_2 of 40

c. Set what you are going to change, and set it equal to x (Rate $= x$ or $V_T = x$). It is easier to change the rate.

   $1000 \text{ V}_T \times \text{Rate } 10 \times 60 \text{ CO}_2 = 1000 \text{ V}_T \times \text{Rate } x \times 40 \text{ CO}_2$

d. Solve by algebra for x. This gives you an estimate of the amount of change.

   $600 = 40x$
   $15 = x$
   Now change the rate to 15.

e. Obtain an ABG 20 minutes after the change to evaluate the difference that the change made.

3. One can change the tidal volume instead of the rate if one so desires. Just solve for the tidal volume of the desired change.

4. Do not "shoot from the hip" when it comes to giving HCO_3 or making ventilator changes. These tools allow accurate diagnosis and treatment. Check an ABG 20 minutes after an intervention.

EXAMPLE: A classic ABG would be 7.30/35/65.
a. Patient is "down" 5, and so should be "up" 0.04 (or rather "4"). The predicted pH is 7.44. But it is not. There is a difference in the predicted and the measured pH.
b. (7.44 predicted − 7.30 measured) = 0.14 (i.e., 14).

c. $14 \times \frac{2}{3} = 9.3$. The measured pH is more acidic than predicted. The patient has a base deficit of 9.

This patient is in *BIG TROUBLE*. He is "making" lots of acid. Note that the values are within the "normal" range and would not even "light up" on most ABG panels. This is the reason one computes the base deficit each time ABG results are received.

The patient has a metabolic acidosis. Compute how much HCO_3 to give him (the patient weighs 70 kg):

$$0.4 \text{ Bicarbonate space} \times 70 \text{ kg} \times 9 \text{ Base deficit} =$$
$$252 \text{ mEq } HCO_3 \text{ needed in his bicarbonate space}$$

Remember: Give only half that value, 126 mEq, or 2.5 ampules of HCO_3 now, then check another ABG in 20 minutes. Search for a cause.

Evaluation of Oxygenation

The patient has a PO_2 of 65. This should reflect a saturation of 94%. This is not a problem at this time. The PO_2 may look "low"; however, one needs to remember the hemoglobin-oxygen dissociation curve.

SOME USEFUL VENTILATORY EQUATIONS
A-a Gradient Equation

1. The alveolar-arterial gradient (A-a gradient) or A-a O_2 difference ($DA-aO_2$) is the difference between the partial pressure of oxygen in alveoli (A) and that in arterial blood (a):

$$DA-aO_2 = PAO_2 - PaO_2$$

a. $DA-aO_2$ is 5 to 15 in normal young patients.
b. $DA-aO_2$ is increased in all causes of hypoxemia except hypoventilation and high altitude. It increases with age and is increased in patients with lung diseases that cause a V/Q mismatch (i.e., shunt or diffusion abnormality). A patient with a

pulmonary embolus has an increased $DA\text{-}aO_2$, but if the patient is hyperventilating (as is often the case), the ABG may show a normal PaO_2.

c. To determine the $DA\text{-}aO_2$, first determine the PaO_2 in the alveoli (PAO_2). This is the partial pressure of inspired O_2 minus the partial pressure of alveolar CO_2 ($PACO_2$). The $PACO_2 = PaCO_2/0.8$. The 0.8 used in this short formula represents the *respiratory quotient* (CO_2 produced per minute or O_2 consumed per minute). Note that the partial pressure of CO_2 in the alveoli is slightly lower than in arterial blood.

$$PAO_2 = \text{Inspired } PaO_2 - (PaCO_2 \div 0.8)$$

d. The inspired PaO_2 is determined by multiplying the $\%O_2$ (same as the FIO_2) × (Barometric pressure − Water vapor). At standard conditions barometric pressure = 760 mm Hg and water vapor = 47 mm Hg. Plugging this back into the original formula gives:

$$DA\text{-}aO_2 = PAO_2 - PaO_2$$
$$DA\text{-}aO_2 = [FIO_2 \times (\text{Barometric pressure} - $$
$$\text{Water vapor pressure}) - (PaCO_2 \div 0.8)] - PaO_2$$

Assuming standard conditions (often unlikely), the equation would be:

$$DA\text{-}aO_2 = [0.21 \times (760 - 47) - (PaCO_2 \div 0.8)] - PaO_2$$
$$DA\text{-}aO_2 = [150 - (PaCO_2 \div 0.8)] - PaO_2$$

e. This calculation is most accurate at an FIO_2 of 0.21.
At an FIO_2 of 0.21, normal is 10-20 mm Hg; >25 is abnormal.
At an FIO_2 of 1.00, >350 is abnormal.

2. Another method to calculate this mentally at the bedside is as follows.

    a. The A-a gradient is: $DA\text{-}aO_2 = 150 - (PaO_2 + 1.25\ PaCO_2)$

    b. $DA\text{-}aO_2$ increases with age. Two rules of thumb for determining normal $DA\text{-}aO_2$ are:

- Normal $DA\text{-}aO_2$ is less than or equal to 0.29 (age).

      or

- Normal $DA\text{-}aO_2$ is less than or equal to (age $\div$ 4) + 2.5.

3. Yet another bedside calculation is as follows.

    a. The A-a gradient is: $700 \times FIO_2 - PCO_2$

    b. Abnormal is >300. *(Consider intubation.)*

    c. PAO_2 = Alveolar air pressure of O_2. PaO_2 = arterial air pressure of O_2. PCO_2 = Arterial air pressure of CO_2. FIO_2 = Fractional inspired oxygen. PB + Barometric pressure (usually 740 mm Hg at sea level). R = Respiratory quotient = CO_2/O_2 of expired air.

4. Respiratory causes of an increased A-a gradient include diffusion barrier, right to left intrapulmonary shunt, and V/Q mismatch. Nonrespiratory causes include; right to left intracardiac shunts and hyperthermia. A decreased PaO_2 with a normal A-a gradient is seen at high altitude, with a decreased respiratory quotient, and in central hypoventilation.

Compliance Equation

1. $C = \Delta V/\Delta P$.

2. $C_{dyn} = VT/$Peak transpulmonary pressure. This measures the compliance during movement of air. Desired is <0.3 cm H_2O/sec.

3. $C_{stat} = VT/$Plateau pressure = 1/Elastic recoil. This measures the compliance at end expiration when there is no air flow. Included is the compliance of the chest wall. Normal = 0.05 − 0.07 L/cm H_2O.

REFERENCES

1. Purdue GF, Hunt JL. Inhalation injuries and burns in the inner city. Surg Clin North Am 7(2):385-397, 1991.

2. Rue LW III, Cioffi WG, Mason AD, McManus WF, Pruitt BA Jr. Improved survival of burned patients with inhalation injury. Arch Surg 128:772-778, 1993.

3. Demling R, Picard L, Campbell C, Lalonde C. Relationship of burn induced lung lipid peroxidation of the degree of injury after smoke inhalation and a body burn. Crit Care Med 21:1935-1943, 1993.

4. Valova M, Konigova R, Broz L, Zajicek R, Toupalik P. Early and late fatal complications of inhalation injury. Acta Chir Plast 44(2):51-54, 2002.

5. Einhorn IN. Physiological and toxicological aspects of smoke produced during the combustion of polymeric materials. Environ Health Perspect 11:163-189, 1975.

6. Schulte JH. Effects of mild carbon monoxide intoxication. Arch Environ Health 7:524-530, 1963.

7. Holm C, Tegeler J, Mayr M, Pfeiffer U, Henckel von Donnersmarck G, Muhlbauer W. Effect of crystalloid resuscitation and inhalation injury on extravascular lung water: Clinical implications. Chest 121(6):1956-1962, 2002.

8. Pulmonary physiology and disease in the burn patient. ABA Postgraduate course. Chicago: American Burn Association, 1996.

9. Saab M, Majid I. Acute pulmonary oedema following smoke inhalation. I. Int J Clin Pract 54(2):115-116, 2000.

10. Barillo DJ, Goode R, Esch V. Cyanide poisoning in victims of fire: Analysis of 364 cases and review of the literature. J Burn Care Rehabil 15:46-51, 1994.

11. Nakae H, Tanaka H, Inaba H. Failure to clear casts and secretions following inhalation injury can be dangerous: Report of a case. Burns 27(2):189-191, 2001.

12. Heimbach DM, Waeckerle JF. Inhalation injuries. Ann Emerg Med 17:1316-1323, 1988.

13. Whitman GJR. Resident's Manual Cardiac Surgery Service. Philadelphia: Medical College of Pennsylvania, 1994.

14. Derdak S. High frequency oscillatory ventilation for accurate respiratory distress syndrome in adult patients. Crit Care Med 31(4):S317-323, 2003.

7 ▪ General (Nonburn) Inpatient Wound Care

THE BASICS

There are a few general principles that the practitioner caring for wounds should know, including knowledge of the phases of wound healing, the entities that must be present, and what entities can hamper wound healing.

In this chapter we will discuss care of common wounds as well as more complex wounds that the practitioner will see as he or she treats inpatients.

STAGES OF WOUND HEALING

The process of wound healing may be broken down into various phases. These phases are influenced by the dominant cellular type in the wound site. The phases and cell types may overlap. After the integrity of the skin is disrupted, vasoconstriction occurs and a platelet plug is formed. Platelets are essential for hemostasis; they also activate other cells and start the inflammatory cascade. The wound-healing process begins with the inflammatory response. The wound site swells, vasodilation occurs, and the reaction is mediated by multiple cytokines, growth factors, and local proteins. Some of these molecules (called *chemoattractants*) attract other cells to the wound. Leukocytes appear quickly in the wound and mediate bacterial phagocytosis and lysis. They predominate from the time of wounding until about day 3. The monocyte is next to appear; it is the key mediator of the cellular response within the wound. Fibrinogen appears to aid in adherence of the wound edges. Histamine, prostaglandins, and vasoactive substances mediate hemostasis. This phase of healing is called the *lag, substrate,* or *inflammatory phase.* This phase must occur to prepare the wound for the subsequent phases of healing. The monocyte is the predominant cell from days 3 to 7.

The second phase of wound healing is the *fibroblastic* or *collagen phase.* Fibroblasts begin to proliferate and prepare for their important role of collagen synthesis. As the collagen content increases, the wound strengthens. The wound's tensile strength and collagen content increase over the next few weeks. The maximum collagen content is in the wound at 6 weeks after injury. The fibroblasts are the predominant cells in the wound. Most modeling is done by 1 year; collagen turnover within the wound will continue indefinitely. The maximum bursting strength of the wound will never reach that of undamaged skin but will usually achieve 80%. This is achieved at 6 months after the wound occurred.

Cofactors are important in proper collagen formation and wound healing. Ascorbic acid (vitamin C) is essential for collagen formation. Without vitamin C, proline cannot be hydroxylated to hydroxyproline, and collagen synthesis stops. Collagen resorption will continue at a normal pace, leading to scurvy. In 1747 Dr. James Lind, a surgeon in the British navy, discovered that by giving sailors limes and other citrus fruits to eat, they did not develop scurvy, thus helping to make sailors on long voyages fit for duty and earning them the nickname "limeys."

The third and final phase of wound healing also lasts the longest. This is the *maturation* or *remodeling phase.* This phase may continue for several years. Progressive collagen replacement allows scars to flatten out and become paler with time. Most surgeons will not revise a scar until at least 9 months to 1 year after the initial injury; by that time the collagen content and remodeling usually have stabilized.[1,2]

WOUNDS WITH LOSS OF SKIN

Acute, traumatic injuries (a full-thickness burn, a deep abrasion, or an avulsion injury) will pass through the same phases of wound healing. In such an injury the closure and healing is more complex, requiring additional mechanisms.

Epithelial proliferation and migration are required for healing of the wound. This process starts after the biochemical and cellular milieu is ready, and bacterial contamination of the wound is below 10^5 organisms per cubic centimeter of tissue. If the wound is superficial, the epithelium can spread from the sweat glands and hair follicles as well as the wound edges to cover the wound. Depending on its size, the wound may be covered in this fashion in 10 to 14 days. In full-thickness wounds epithelium migrates from the wound margins. This epithelization is a slow process, with migration approximately 1 mm/day. Epithelium is also more susceptible to injury, because it migrates without an accompanying dermal layer. Histologically, migratory epithelium often appears neoplastic. Indeed, a chronic wound not closed for many years may become a malignant ulcer, or *Marjolin's ulcer* (named for the French surgeon Marjolin, who first described this entity). Therefore one cannot wait for epithelialization to heal the wound alone, except in very small or superficial injuries. In these cases, grafts and flaps are used to cover the wound.

Wound contraction is another important entity in the closure of these types of wounds. The surface fills with granulation tissue. This tissue consists of capillary and fibroblast proliferation. After granulation, myofibroblasts, behaving like smooth muscle cells, mediate the contraction of the wound. This process may lead to contractures. Contraction may be slowed by the application of split-thickness skin grafts and may be almost stopped with placement of a full-thickness skin graft. Contamination of the wound will stop both epithelialization and contraction of the wound.[1,2]

WOUND CONTAMINATION

Contamination of the wound may hamper or halt the healing process. A wound is much more susceptible to infection and breakdown than intact skin is. The objective in the decontamination of wounds is to reduce the bacterial count to less than 10^5 organisms per cubic centimeter of tissue. This can be accomplished with the use of debridement of necrotic or infected tissue, and irrigation. Normal saline solution is the irrigant of choice. Use of a sedative, analgesia, and a local anesthetic is highly recommended. Some cases (e.g., "road rash" after a motorcycle motor vehicle accident [MVA]) may require general anesthesia for adequate debridement and irrigation. Remember to ask the patient about drug reactions and allergies. Reassurance and explanation of the procedure will also help the patient during the process.[3]

DECUBITUS ULCERS

Decubitus ulcers form because of a lack of oxygen and/or nutrient materials to meet the needs of the tissue. They are usually caused by pressure exerted on an area of tissue, not allowing adequate perfusion. These wounds may occur rapidly; indeed, only 2 hours may be required for the formation of such a wound.

The principles of treatment correspond to those mentioned previously. These include good nutrition, adequate blood flow, relief from continuous pressure, and decontamination of the wound. Inpatients who do not have the capacity to move themselves should be turned every few hours, and their skin should be inspected for signs of early breakdown. Special mattresses have been devised to this end. Criteria for use of these beds have been determined (Box 7-1).

The principles of debridement of these wounds were discussed earlier. Sharp debridement of necrotic, infected, or fibrous tissue may be necessary. This usually can be performed at the patient's bedside. Debridement with the use of dressings may be appropriate in

Box 7-1
Criteria for Selection of Pressure Reduction/Relief Devices

I. Continuous airflow—wound care committee approval required; high-risk patient with no skin breakdown.

II. Low air loss—wound care committee approval required.
   A. General health—critical; major surgery with chronic/serious health problems; major/multiple injury. Rehabilitative phase; patients whose respiratory status requires high head elevation.
   B. Mental status—comatose; minimal/no verbal response; minimal/no motor response to painful stimuli.
   C. Activity—patients requiring transfer; completely bedridden.
   D. Mobility—very limited or immobile; minimal voluntary movement/positioning.
   E. Elimination—frequent/complete loss of bowel and bladder control; signs of maceration due to exposure to urine/feces.
   F. Nutrition—consumes <50% of recommended diet; orally or intravenously only; albumin <2.5 g/dl.
   G. Skin integrity—stage 2; noninfected stages 3 and 4.

III. Air fluidized—wound care committee approval required.
   A. General health—critical; major surgery with chronic/serious health problems; major/multiple injuries. Burn patients; patients with skin grafts, flaps, donor sites; multiple trauma in acute phase.
   B. Mental status—comatose; minimal/no verbal response; minimal/no motor response to painful stimuli.
   C. Activity—completely bedridden.
   D. Mobility—immobile; minimal to no voluntary movement/positioning.
   E. Elimination—frequent/complete loss of bowel and bladder control; signs of maceration due to exposure to urine/feces.
   F. Nutrition—consumes <50% of recommended diet; orally or intravenously only; albumin <2.5 g/dl.
   G. Skin integrity—complicated stage 2; stages 3 and 4 and multiple pressure sores.

From Granick MS, Solomon MP, Wind S, Goldberg M. Wound care and wound management. Adv Plast Reconstr Surg 12:110, 1996. (Reprinted with permission from Mosby–Year Book.)
A modified Norton scale bed is indicated when one or more apply when individual patient treatment objectives are considered.

some cases to keep the wound clean. Wet-to-dry dressings with normal saline solution, changed three times per day, will debride small amounts of material. Dakin's solution, or a 1:1000 mixture of povidone-iodine and saline, or 0.5% acetic acid in saline solution may be used if bacterial overgrowth is suspected. Do not apply wet dressings to nonwounded skin.

Table 7-1 is a guide to wound care objectives and the products used to achieve these objectives. Granulation tissue may occasionally hamper the epithelialization process. Use of silver nitrate sticks can decrease the amount of granulation tissue to allow epithelialization.

Negative pressure devices can be useful in many cases to help contract the wound as well as keep it clean. Fewer dressing changes are involved, thus easing the burden on the nursing staff and the patient. This modality allows treatment of the wound while improving the patient's nutritional status. It may lessen the size of the wound and therefore change the choice of surgical coverage to a less sophisticated one.[4] This is becoming the modality of choice in most instances. It also allows time for nutritional support to be given to the patient for wound healing.

Myocutaneous flaps and skin grafts are appropriate in selected patients.[5] In one series[6] it was seen that a multidisciplinary wound care team was instrumental in the lowering of the incidence and length of healing of these wounds.

INFECTED WOUNDS

These wounds should be left open until contamination and infection is controlled and the normal wound healing process can commence. Identification and treatment of the infectious cause depends on appropriate antibiotics, irrigation, and debridement to resolve the problem. Myocutaneous flaps may be used in some cases to bring coverage and blood supply to the debrided area.

Text continued on p. 96.

Table 7-1. Wound care products by objective

Wound care objective	Product		Function	Outcome	Cautions	Example (manufacturer)
	Category					
Cleansing						
Skin	Liquid/foam skin		Emulsifies waste materials, neutralizes drainage and odors	Facilitates the removal of surface debris	Use *around* wounds, not for use *in* wounds	Perineal Cleansing Foam (Carrington) Periwash (Sween Inc.) Triple Care (Smith & Nephew)
Wound	Absorbent foam					
		Hydrophilic-hydrophobic	Absorption of minimal to heavy exudate, nonadherent	Nonadherent, decreased tissue trauma on removal	Affixed by external dressing, do not allow to dry out	Allevyn (Smith & Nephew) Epi-Lock (Calgon Vestal) Lyofoam (Acme)
	Gels		Absorb minimal to heavy exudate, soften necrotic tissue, nonadherent	Conforms to wound surface, eliminates dead space, moist environment	Requires cover dressing, replace as needed to keep wound base moist	Absorption Dressing (Bard) Intrasite (Smith & Nephew) Hypergel (Scott Health Care)
	Hydrogels		Absorb minimal exudate, nonadherent, may soften necrosis	Creates moist environment, soothes and protects	Do not allow to dry out, may require cover dressing to hold in place	Aquasorb (DeRoyal Industries) Nu-Gel (Johnson & Johnson) Vigilon (Bard)

From Granick MS, Solomon MP, Wind S, Goldberg M. Wound care and wound management. Adv Plast Reconstr Surg 12:99-121, 1996. (Reprinted with permission from Mosby–Year Book.)

Continued.

Table 7-1. Wound care products by objective—cont'd

Wound care objective	Product			Outcome	Cautions	Example (manufacturer)
	Category	Function				
Cleansing—cont'd						
Wound—cont'd	Normal saline solution, sprays	Mechanical cleansing action—sometimes used to "wet" dressings		Surface debris removal without wound irritation	Do not apply with excessive force	Dermal Wound Cleansers (Smith & Nephew) Puri Clens (Sween Inc.) Shur-Clens (Calgon Vestal)
	Impregnated gauze Crystalline sodium chloride dressing	Osmotic action "wicks" exudate from wound and surrounding tissue		Cleanses and reduces edema, retards bacterial growth	Cover with dry dressing to absorb exudate	Mesalt (Scott Health Care)
Autolytic	Hydrocolloids	Occlusion traps exudate, facilitating white blood cells to liquefy and phagocytize necrosis		Selective (specific) debridement, some absorption of exudate	Never use on any wound suspected of being infected	Duoderm (ConvaTec; Squibb) Restore (Hollister) Replicare (Smith & Nephew) Tegasorb (3M)
	Hydrogels	Moisture helps soften eschar in dry, necrotic wounds		Softens and aids removal of eschar	Held in place by external dressing, do not allow to dry out	Aquasorb (DeRoyal Industries) Hypergel (Scott Health Care) Nu-Gel (Johnson & Johnson) SoloSite (Smith & Nephew)

	MVP films, semi-occlusive	Acts as occlusive, also allows the exchange of gases, vapors	Selective debridement	Bioclusive (Johnson & Johnson) OpSite (Smith & Nephew; United) Tegaderm (3M)
Chemical	Enzymes	Chemically digest debris and necrotic tissue	Nonselective (nonspecific) debridement	Do not us on infected wounds Cross hatch eschar, protect periwound; iodine renders some ineffective	Collagenase (Biozyme C) Fibrinolysin (Elase) Streptokinase (Varidase) Sutilains (Travase; Flint)
Mechanical	Impregnated gauze Crystalline sodium chloride dressing	Creates hypertonic environment, "wicks" bacteria, softens necrotic tissue	Selective debridement	Cover with dry dressings to absorb exudate	Mesalt (Scott Health Care)
	Surgical	Dissection	Selective debridement	Wound increases in size	
	Wet-to-dry	Plain gauze traps wound debris	Nonselective debridement	Not for patients with bleeding problems	Nu-Brede (Johnson & Johnson)
	Whirlpool/irrigations	Mechanical removal of debris, necrosis	Nonselective debridement	Force rather than solution gives results	

Continued.

Table 7-1. Wound care products by objective—cont'd

Wound care objective	Product		Outcome	Cautions	Example (manufacturer)
	Category	Function			
Protection					
Skin	Creams, lotions, ointments, sprays	Lubricates, softens, some form occlusive barrier	Rehydration and/or protection	Predominantly used on intact skin	Moisture Barrier Ointment (Carrington) Pericare (Sween Inc.) Triple Care (Smith & Nephew) Uni-salve (Smith & Nephew) Allkare (ConvaTec; Squibb) Incontinence Barrier Film (Bard)
	Skin sealants	Forms layer of plastic polymer over skin	Protection from corrosive drainage and friction of tape removal	May contain varying amounts of alcohol that stings denuded skin	Skin Gel (Hollister) Skin Prep (Smith & Nephew)
Wound	MVP films, semiocclusive	Forms semiocclusive seal over wound	Protection, moist wound base	*Never* use on infected wound	Bioclusive (Johnson & Johnson) OpSite (Smith & Nephew) Tegaderm (3M)
	Foam dressings, semiocclusive	Forms semiocclusive seal over wound; reportedly maintains wound temperature	Protection, moist wound base	Must be affixed by external dressing	Allevyn (Smith & Nephew) Epi-Lock (Calgon Vestal) Lyofoam (Acme; United)

Gelatin/pectin wafers (occlusive)	Forms occlusive seal, absorbs skin moisture to prevent maceration	Protection, moist wound base	*Never* use on infected wound	Premium Barrier (Hollister) Stomahesive (ConvaTec; Squibb) Sween-A-Peel (Sween Inc.)
Hydrocolloids (occlusive)	As gelatin, forms gel over wound bed to decrease trauma of removal	Protection, moist wound base, less removal trauma	*Never* use on infected wound	DuoDerm (ConvaTec; Squibb) Replicare (Smith & Nephew) Restore (Hollister) Tegasorb (3M)
Ointments, gels	Provides protective, moist environment	Moist wound base	Reapply often to maintain moist environment	Biolex Wound Gel (Catalina) Dermal Wound Gel (Carrington) Dermagram (Dermasciences)

TISSUE DAMAGE FROM RADIATION THERAPY

Radiation therapy can be an important adjunct in the treatment of cancer. Radiation kills tumor cells—but also damages normal surrounding tissues. The amount of injury depends on the cell's susceptibility to radiation, its stage in the growth cycle, and its growth rate. Radiation damage to the skin in the acute phase is secondary to an inflammatory reaction, causing the skin to be dry, erythematous, and scaly. These acute changes will usually resolve within 6 months. Chronic changes that appear later (beyond 6 months) are atrophy, edema, hyperpigmentation or hypopigmentation, fissuring, brittleness, and telangiectasias. Delayed complications of radiation therapy include spontaneous necrosis, inability of wounds to heal, alteration of the local blood supply, fibrosis, and secondary tumors.[7]

Radiation therapy is reported to have its maximal effect on wound healing when given within 2 weeks of surgery. Injury to fibroblasts and endothelial cells and decreased collagen production are thought to account for some of the mechanisms causing impaired wound healing. Fibrosis of blood vessels leading to impaired perfusion, and subsequent lower percutaneous oxygen tension within the wound tissue has also been implicated. Some suggest that radiation therapy be withheld until 2 to 3 weeks after surgery, at which point initial wound healing may be completed.[8]

When a patient develops skin breakdown within a zone of radiation tissue, a biopsy must be performed to rule out tumor recurrence or secondary tumor. Local management of the wound requires aggressive debridement of all devitalized tissue, including skeletal support when necessary. Vascularized nonirradiated tissue is required for adequate reconstruction.[5]

CHEMOTHERAPY

It has been shown that it may be prudent to delay chemotherapy until 7 to 10 days after surgery.[9] Many products of oncogenes are similar, if not identical, to growth factors. Many schemas of cancerous replication are similar to those in wound repair. The chemotherapeutic agents may hamper growth factors and other mechanisms engaged in healing the wound. The use of topical growth factors is contraindicated in most cancerous wounds.[10]

LEG ULCERATIONS

Chronic venous disease is a prominent cause of leg ulcers. Venous ulcerations can also be caused by phlebitic syndromes, chronic venous stasis, and deep venous thrombosis. Venous ulcers are typically located on the medial malleolar area and are usually superficial with a good bed of granulation tissue. The limbs are often edematous and indurated, with considerable chronic skin atrophy.

Patients with diabetes frequently develop distal neuropathies that lead to ulceration. Their altered sensation can allow ulcers on the lower extremities to go unnoticed until the wounds become advanced. In addition, these wounds often become secondarily infected.

Peripheral vascular disease (PVD) of the lower extremities is a known risk factor for delayed wound healing, with increasing propensity for ulceration, infection, and gangrene. Associated risk factors for PVD include those that lead to atherosclerosis (e.g., cigarette smoking, hypertension, hyperlipidemia, and diabetes mellitus).

Less commonly, leg ulcerations may result from other diseases, such as rheumatoid arthritis, ankylosing spondylitis, sickle cell disease, or be the result of an underlying squamous or basal cell carcinoma.

Treatment of leg ulcers depends on an adequate blood supply. Once this has been ensured by medical treatment (with appropriate medicines) or surgical modalities (i.e., vascular bypass) and the patient's status has been medically optimized (i.e., cardiopulmonary maximization and/or negative pressure application to the wound), reconstruction with the use of grafts or flaps can be considered if necessary.[5,8,11]

REFERENCES

1. Verheyden CN, Losee J, Miller MJ, Rockwell WB, Slezak S, eds. Plastic and Reconstructive Surgery: Essentials for Students, 6th ed. Arlington Heights, Ill: Plastic Surgery Educational Foundation, 2002.

2. Simmons RL, Steed DL. Wound healing. In Simmons RL, Steed DL, Simmons J, eds. Basic Science Review for Surgeons. Philadelphia: WB Saunders, 1992.

3. Fisher JC, Achauer BM, Brody GS, Frank DH, Noone RB, Robson MC, Smoot W III, Thorne FL. Everyday Wounds: A Guide for the Primary Care Physician. Arlington Heights, Ill: Plastic Surgery Educational Foundation, 1997.

4. Ford CN, Reinhard ER, Yeh D, Syrek D, De Las Morenas A, Bergman SB, Williams S, Hamori CA. Interim analysis of a prospective, randomized trial of vacuum-assisted closure versus the healthpoint system in the management of pressure ulcers. Ann Plast Surg 49(1):55-61, 2002.

5. Foster RD, Anthony JP, Mathes SJ, Hoffman WY, Young D, Eshima I. Flap selection as a determinant of success in pressure sore coverage. Arch Surg 132(8):868-873, 1997.

6. Granick MS, Solomon MP, Wind S, Goldberg M. Wound management and wound care. Adv Plast Reconstr Surg 12:99-121, 1996.

7. Mendelsohn FA, Divino CM, Reis ED, Kerstein MD. Wound care after radiation therapy. Adv Skin Wound Care 15(5):216-224, 2002.

8. McCaw DL. The effects of cancer and cancer therapies on wound healing. Semin Vet Med Surg Small Anim 4:281-286, 1989.

9. Falcone RE, Nappi JF. Chemotherapy and wound healing. Surg Clin North Am 64:779-794, 1984.

10. Roth JJ, Albo D, Rothman VL, Longaker MT, Granick MS, Long CD, Solomon MP, Tuszynski GP. Thrombospondin-1 and its CSVTCG-specific receptor in wound healing and cancer. Ann Plast Surg 40(5):494-501, 1998.

11. Lau HC, Granick MS, Aisner AM, Solomon MP. Wound care in the elderly patient. In Surgery in the Elderly Patient II. Surg Clin North Am 74(2):441-463, 1994.

8 ■ Toxic Epidermal Necrolysis Syndrome

Toxic epidermal necrolysis syndrome (TENS) presents as sloughing of the skin. There are a few variations of this disease. The causes vary as well. TENS type 1 (staphylococcal scalded skin syndrome [SSSS]) is usually caused by a staphylococcal toxin. This occurs most commonly in children and has a mortality rate of 5% or less. The toxin causes epidermis separation at the subgranular intraepidermal plane. This entity, although rare, can occur in children after initial burn care.

TENS type 2 is clinically a variant of erythema multiforme major. Adults are more commonly affected. The mortality rate is estimated to be 25% to 50%. Histologic examination shows cleavage at the dermal-epidermal junction. It is often difficult to distinguish TENS 1 (SSSS) from TENS 2 clinically, but histologic examination of the denuded skin can assist in distinguishing the types. TENS 1 will have only the stratum corneum denuded, whereas TENS 2 will show the entire epidermis sloughed. Stevens-Johnson syndrome is TENS type 2 with internal organ involvement.

TENS 2 is a drug-induced, dose-independent reaction. The sulfonamides and phenytoin are the most common etiologic agents.[1] The period between administration of the drug and development of TENS is between 1 and 3 weeks. However, phenytoin can take up to 8 weeks to cause TENS. If the patient has had a previous reaction to the drug, the time period can be as short as 2 days. In addition to drugs, several viruses and malignancies have been implicated.

The pathophysiology of TENS remains poorly understood. One hypothesis is TENS has an immunologic cause, because monocellular infiltrates are often detected in the dermis. Lymphokine involvement may also mediate the epidermal injury.

The clinical presentation of TENS begins with a prodrome of fever and other symptoms that resemble an upper respiratory tract infection. This can continue for 1 to 3 weeks before cutaneous involvement is noted. The patient demonstrates fever and sloughing of the epidermis and mucous membranes. This acute cutaneous phase can last for 1 to 2 weeks. Urticarial plaques are typically present; these progress to bullae and coalesce. The fluid within them is clear, yellow, and acellular. The epidermis will slough in large sheets, leaving a denuded dermis (Nikolsky's sign). One in seven patients will experience a 100% loss of epidermis. The only area that appears to escape this process is the scalp. Any epidermal surface can be involved, including the conjunctiva and the gastrointestinal tract (including the gallbladder and pancreas). Less commonly, the disease can involve the respiratory tract and the vaginal membranes. Recovery time is usually 1 to 2 weeks. TENS injury typically heals more rapidly than burned skin. The healing process is slowed by infection, trauma, and pressure.

TENS carries a high morbidity rate. This can be secondary to respiratory or renal failure, gastrointestinal bleeding, pulmonary embolism, and sepsis.[2] Mortality rates are also significant; sepsis is the most common cause of death in TENS patients. *Pseudomonas* and *Staphylococcus* are the most common organisms identified.

A large prospective study recently stated that erythema multiforme major differs from Stevens-Johnson syndrome and toxic epidermal necrolysis not only in severity, but also in several demographic characteristics and causes. Erythema multiforme presents with an increased occurrence in younger males, less fever, more frequent recurrences, and milder mucosal lesions. Erythema multiforme does not seem to be associated with collagen vascular diseases, HIV infection, or cancer. Recent or recurrent herpes was the principal risk factor for erythema multiforme major (29% and 17%, respectively), and had a role in Stevens-Johnson syndrome (6% and 10%, respectively), but not toxic epidermal necrolysis. Drugs were found to be a more common cause of Stevens-Johnson syndrome and toxic epidermal necrolysis (64% to 66%) than of erythema multiforme major (18%).[3]

TREATMENT

The burn center is an ideal place for the treatment of TENS patients.[1,4,5] Staff members are well trained and comfortable with treating patients with massive cutaneous injuries and the concomitant systemic effects. The physical plant is also conducive to the treatment and comfort of these patients.

On admission to the burn unit, steroid medications are discontinued because of the increased morbidity and mortality rate associated with their use. Systemic antibiotics are also discontinued if there are no signs of sepsis or documented infection. Indwelling catheters are removed or changed. Fluid resuscitation is important. Less fluid is needed than is typical in burn resuscitation, because there is less edema formation in TENS.

Loose epidermis is removed by the burn team, and a biopsy is performed to confirm the diagnosis. Porcine xenografts are used for coverage. Bacitracin is used for coverage on the face; silver nitrate is used on areas not covered by xenografts. Silver sulfadiazine and mafinide are not used, because they have been known to cause TENS.

TENS can permanently damage vision. Ophthalmology should be consulted early in the course of the TENS patient. Antibiotic solutions are used to treat the conjunctivitis. Adhesions may also form on the conjunctival surfaces. These should be brushed aside with a glass rod, up to four times per day, to avoid immobilization. Warm compresses and rinses with saline solution may relieve discomfort. Photophobia is relieved by wearing dark glasses.

Nutrition is important in the treatment of these patients. There is nitrogen loss and an increased metabolic rate. Usually, 2500 Kcal/day will provide sufficient calories. This is a starting point. The patient's nutritional status should be monitored as discussed in previous chapters. Enteral feeding is the preferred route if the patient can tolerate it. Procalamine can be used to augment the patient's intake via a peripheral intravenous line. If this is not sufficient, one should consider initiating TPN via a central line.

Improved treatment techniques and critical care have decreased the mortality and morbidity of this disease. Prompt recognition of the disease and admission of the patient to an appropriate care center, the burn unit, with its aforementioned attributes, has aided in the treatment of adults and children.[6-9]

Research continues into the pathophysiology and treatment of this disease. One promising treatment is the use of immunoglobulin for the treatment of TENS.

REFERENCES

1. Kelemem JJ III, Cioffi WG, McManus WF, Mason AD Jr, Pruitt BA Jr. Burn center care for patients with toxic epidermal necrolysis. J Am Coll Surg 180(3): 273-278, 1995.
2. Revuz J, Penson D, Roujeau JC, Cuillaume JC, Payne CR, Wechsler J, Touraine R. Toxic epidermal necrolysis: Clinical findings and prognostic factors in 87 patients. Arch Dermatol 123(9):1156-1158, 1987.
3. Auquier-Dunant A, Mockenhaupt M, Naldi L, Correia O, Schroder W, Roujeau JC. Correlations between clinical patterns and causes of erythema multiforme majus, Stevens-Johnson syndrome, and toxic epidermal necrolysis: Results of an international prospective study. Arch Dermatol 138(8):1019-1024, 2002.
4. Halebian PH, Corder VJ, Madden MR, Finklestein JL, Shires GT. Improved burn center survival of patients with toxic epidermal necrolysis managed without corticosteroids. Ann Surg 204(5):503-512, 1986.

5. Taylor JA, Globe B, Heinbach GM, Bergman AB. Toxic epidermal necrolysis. A comprehensive approach. Multidisciplinary management in a burn center. Clin Pediatr 28(9):404-407, 1989.
6. Ducic I, Shalom A, Rising W, Nagamoto K, Munster AM. Outcome of patients with toxic epidermal necrolysis syndrome revisited. Plast Reconstr Surg 110(3):768-773, 2002.
7. Heimbach DM, Engrav LH, Marvin JA, Hamar TJ, Grube BJ. Toxic epidermal necrolysis: A step forward in treatment. JAMA 257(16):2171-2175, 1987.
8. Sheridan RL, Schulz JT, Ryan CM, Schnitzer JJ, Lawlor D, Driscoll DN, Donelan MB, Tompkins RG. Long-term consequences of toxic epidermal necrolysis in children. Pediatrics 109(1):74-78, 2002.
9. Spies M, Sanford AP, Aili Low JF, Wolf SE, Herndon DN. Treatment of extensive toxic epidermal necrolysis in children. Pediatrics 108(5):1162-1168, 2001.

9 ▪ Electrical Burns

Electrical burns are a unique mechanism of traumatic injury. The extent of damage is usually associated with voltage, type of current, resistance of the tissue, and duration of contact. Electrical burns account for 5% to 10% of burn unit admissions but are responsible for a disproportionate amount of morbidity and mortality.[1-3] The number of accidents and deaths related to electricity is on the decline.[4] The main causes of injury include misuse of electrical appliances, inattentiveness, lack of education in safety precautions, and lack of parental supervision.[5] Approximately 81% are occupation-related injuries.[3]

Electrical energy is converted to heat, causing thermal injury. Heat generation depends on the strength of the current, duration of flow, and resistance of the tissue. Increased heat is generated when any of the three is increased. Bone has the highest resistance to current of all tissues, but also is less damaged by heat. Nerves and vessels generate less heat but are easily damaged. Between the entrance and exit points, the current flows in an unpredictable manner. If the skin resistance is high, less current flows through the body. If low resistance is encountered, such as with sweat or when the person is standing in water, more current will flow through the body. Protein is denatured by electrical current, leading to cell death. Blood vessels are occluded, resulting in anoxia and tissue death. Plasma is also lost into the damaged tissue.[6]

Electrical burns are divided into two types: high-voltage and low-voltage burns. High-voltage burns (>1000 volts) usually create more soft tissue damage and are more complex. In addition to the electrical injury, there is an entrance and an exit burn. With high-voltage burns there is the possibility of a thermal burn wound from the flash of the electricity and the ignition of clothing.[7]

Burn percentage is used as a guide for fluid resuscitation. Additional fluid will be necessary if muscle damage is present. If the urine appears clear, the minimum acceptable rate of production is 0.5 ml/kg/hr. A Foley catheter should be used to facilitate appropriate monitoring of urine output. If myoglobin or hemoglobin discoloration is noted, increased urine output is needed to prevent renal failure. A guaiac card may also be used as a bedside check for myoglobinuria. The treatment of myoglobinuria includes mannitol 0.5 mg/kg IV, followed by 1 ampule of bicarbonate IV. IV fluids are increased until the urine is clear. If need be, administration of mannitol and bicarbonate can be repeated if the urine does not clear or if continuing myoglobinuria is suspected. The bicarbonate is used to prevent the precipitation of myoglobin. It is this precipitated myoglobin and its breakdown products that damage the kidney. This damage can lead to renal failure. Acute renal failure occurs in 14.5% of patients. The mortality for patients with renal failure is 59%.[5]

Cardiac abnormalities are another common complication of high-voltage injury. The most common cause of death at the scene is ventricular fibrillation. Myocardial infarction may be a direct result of the injury but carries little risk of reinfarction or hemodynamic consequences. The following patient conditions require cardiac monitoring[8]:

- Cardiac arrest
- Cardiac arrhythmias
- 12-lead ECG abnormalities other than bradycardia or tachycardia
- Loss of consciousness
- Severity of burn or age mandating monitoring

High-voltage burn injury frequently leads to the need for amputation. Deep tissue damage is usually out of proportion to skin damage. Compartment syndrome is also common. Limbs must be frequently checked for swelling, paresthesias, paralysis, pulselessness, pain, and pallor. Pain out of proportion to passive stretch is a sensitive and specific test. Pallor and pulselessness are late signs. With any suspicion of this syndrome, testing of compartment pressures is mandatory. Fasciotomies are the preferred modality of treatment.

High-voltage burns have sequelae throughout subsequent years. Cataracts occur in 5% to 20% of high-voltage burn patients; they may be amenable to surgery and rehabilitation of sight.[9] One third of amputees require stump revision because of heterotopic ossification. Gastrointestinal symptoms include hyperactivity, presenting as vague abdominal complaints and diarrhea. There is also an increased incidence of biliary disease. Neurologic syndromes may appear early or late. In the majority of cases, the motor system is affected and is a spastic rather than a flaccid syndrome. Weakness is a common clinical finding; this can occur in half of electrical injury patients.[10] Significant long-term neurologic deficits can persist in 73 percent of patients (mean follow-up 4.5 years). Only 5.3% of patients after a high-voltage injury were able to return to their preinjury occupation.[1] Therefore it is mandatory that these patients have close, long-term follow-up.

Finally, high-voltage electrical burns are usually obtained at a height (e.g., high-tension lines). If the patient fell during the contact with high voltage, he or she must be treated as a blunt-trauma victim. All trauma must be evaluated as if the patient was not burned. In patients with lightning injuries, a full spine radiographic series should be performed to rule out spinal fractures.

Low-voltage injury can usually be treated conservatively without hospitalizing the patient. These are usually household injuries. The exceptions are severe hand burns and large oral injuries that threaten the airway. For these injuries, neosporin ointment is used twice a day on the lips but not inside the mouth, and if needed, a stretching appliance may be used to restore length and function.

Alternating current presents increased risk of injury because of its tetanic effect. The patient is unable to let go, or break contact with the electrical source, and thus receives further damage from contact. This tetanic contraction of paravertebral muscles, as well as a fall, can result in axial spine fractures.

REFERENCES

1. Hussmann J, Kincan JO, Russell RC, Bradley T, Zamboni WA. Electrical injuries—morbidity, outcome, and treatment rationale. Burns 21(7):530-535, 1995.
2. Xiao J, Cai BR. A clinical study of electrical injuries. Burns 20(4):340-346, 1994.
3. Brandt MM, McReynolds MC, Ahrns KS, Wahl WL. Burn centers should be involved in prevention of occupational electrical injuries. J Burn Care Rehabil 23(2):132-134, 2002.
4. VanDenburg S, McCormik GM II, Young DB. Investigation of deaths related to electrical injury. South Med J 89(9):869-872, 1996.
5. Haberal MA. An eleven-year survey of electrical burn injuries. J Burn Care Rehabil 16(1):43-48, 1995.
6. Fish R. Electric shock. Part I. Physics and pathophysiology. J Emerg Med 11(3):309-312, 1993.
7. Fish R. Electric shock Part II. Nature and mechanisms of injury. J Emerg Med 11(4):457-462, 1993.
8. Hunt JL, Sato R, Baxter C. Acute electric burns. Current diagnostic and therapeutic approaches to management. Arch Surg 115(4):434-438, 1980.
9. Chaudhuri Z, Pandey PK, Bhatia A. Electrical cataract: A case study. Ophthalmic Surg Lasers 33(2):166-168, 2002.
10. Haberal MA, Gurer S, Akman N, Basgoze O. Persistent peripheral nerve pathologies in patients with electrical burns. J Burn Care Rehabil 17(2):147-179, 1996.

10 ▪ Chemical Burns

Chemical burns can occur when a toxic substance is ingested or by direct contact with the skin. Toxic ingestion is commonly seen in suicide attempts by adults and adolescents and occurs accidentally in toddlers. Burns to the skin are commonly seen in industrial workers but may also occur through contact with such mundane household items as alkaline batteries.

INGESTION OF CAUSTICS

Classification of burns of the esophagus is similar to that of burns of the skin. First-degree burn involves the mucosa, with hyperemia, edema, and sloughing. A second-degree burn is transmural. A third-degree burn erodes through the esophagus and involves the peri-esophageal tissue.

Ingestion of detergents and bleach commonly causes only mild esophageal irritation that usually heals without significant morbidity. Acid burns usually cause a coagulation necrosis, which limits its extent. Alkalis produce liquefaction necrosis, in which fat and proteins are saponified and blood vessels thrombose. This leads to further cell death. These factors cause alkalis to penetrate deeply and be resistant to surface irrigation.

Solid alkali substances adhere to the mucosal surfaces and rarely reach the stomach in large enough quantities to neutralize acid. Therefore the burns are typically in the oropharynx and mouth.

These burns are usually distributed in streaks. The mucosa shows areas of white to dark-gray pseudomembranes. The burn produces excessive salivation. Liquid alkali burns all mucosal surfaces. The caustic is usually swallowed, limiting damage to the mouth and pharynx. The major burns are usually to the esophagus and stomach. Reflux pyloric spasm occurs and results in the pooling of the alkali in the stomach. Liquid ingestion burn patients may have odonophagia, dysphagia, and aspiration. They may have retrosternal, back, or peritoneal pain, suggesting mediastinitis or perforation with peritonitis.

TREATMENT

Initially the airway must be surveyed. Intubation may be necessary if there is laryngospasm, edema, or destruction. Intravenous fluid replacement is started. Broad-spectrum antibiotics are started in patients with an esophageal injury. Steroid medications have not been shown to be effective. Because steroids may mask signs of sepsis and peritonitis, we choose not to use them in our unit.

An upper GI radiographic series will demonstrate damaged mucosa, dilation, and perforation. Gastrograffin may be used, although dilute barium will better demonstrate lesions and dilation.

Esophagogastroduodenoscopy (EGD) should be performed after the patient is admitted to grade the injury. A small-caliber pediatric scope will minimize injury. The scope may be advanced carefully beyond the burn, if a burn has a severe portion that is not detected.

First-degree burns can be observed for 24 to 48 hours. The rate of stricture formation in these cases is low. Second- and third-degree burns require close attention. Full-thickness necrosis necessitates excision. Restoration of alimentary continuity should be delayed until recovery from the acute insult has transpired. Second- and third-degree burns typically involve esophageal stricture. Dilation is the mainstay of treatment and should be completed 6 to 8 weeks after injury to minimize perforation. Undilatable strictures require esophageal replacement.

CUTANEOUS CHEMICAL BURNS

Chemicals react with the skin to cause damage from oxidation, reduction, desiccation, and corrosion. Destruction usually occurs with a necrotic central zone surrounded by a peripheral hyperemic zone. In most cases lavaging with water is the most effective immediate therapy, because it washes away the chemical and dilutes the concentration, except as noted in the following discussion.

Alkalis

Alkalis act by dissolving and denaturing proteins. Water is drawn out of the cell and saponification of fat occurs. They also can cause a protein structure to collapse.

Treatment. Rinse with tap water for at least 30 minutes. Ocular injuries should be irrigated with saline solution through a Morgan lens. Topical ophthalmic anesthetics relieve pain and can stop blepharospasm, which will sometimes interfere with copious irrigation of the eye.[1]

Phenols

Phenols are characterized by the substitution of hydrochloral groups for hydrogen groups on a benzene ring. They are found in disinfectants and solvents. These cause skin irritation and can be absorbed cutaneously or inhaled into the lungs. When absorbed, phenols bind to albumin. This can lead to cardiovascular problems (metabolic acidosis, hypertension, ventricular dysrhythmias) and CNS toxicity (coma, seizures), as well as liver failure. Ingestion of as little as 1 g can be fatal; roughly 50% of all reported cases have a fatal outcome. Only a few patients with high serum concentrations after phenol burns have survived.[2] Phenol is not soluble in water. It is excreted in the urine over a 24-hour period.

Treatment. Use copious amounts of pure water,[3] followed by topical application of surgical sponges soaked with polyethylene glycol (PEG). The patient's respiratory and circulatory systems must be stabilized with administration of IV fluid, bicarbonate infusion, and cardiac monitoring. Charcoal should be used for ingestion of a phenol. There are no antidotes, and recovery usually occurs in 1 or 2 days.

Gasoline

An injury from gasoline immersion resembles a small burn. Erythema and blistering are caused by the gasoline's fat-solvent properties. Gasoline contact may cause significant full-thickness burn injuries. Systemic complications may result from the absorption of hydrocarbons through the skin. Regional neuromuscular absorption may produce transient or even permanent impairment.[4] The major injury is pulmonary, including bronchitis, pneumonitis, and pneumonic hemorrhages. Gasoline absorbed into the body is excreted by the pulmonary system.

Treatment. Skin burns should be cleansed and dressed. Burns tend to be superficial and heal spontaneously. There is no antidote.[5,6]

Calcium Oxide

Lime burns are common among concrete workers. Calcium oxide and water (often in the form of sweat), react to form calcium hydroxide, an exothermic reaction. The initial burn under clothing often is not painful. A victim may not know until hours later that he or she has been burned.

Treatment. Lime residue should be brushed away before washing the skin. Remove contaminated clothing. Copiously irrigate the area with water until the soapy feeling has disappeared, then dry the patient thoroughly.

Hydrofluoric Acid

Hydrofluoric acid is used in glassware. It is also seen in some bleach and cleaning agents.[7] It may cause life-threatening hypocalcemia and hypomagnesemia. Hypocalcemia garnered in this manner usually does not show the typical signs. Serum calcium levels and ECG findings will show this hypocalcemia.[8] This hypocalcemia may induce ventricular fibrillation particularly resistant to treatment.[9]

Treatment. The injury is treated by immediate use of 2.5% calcium chloride ointment (usually done while the patient is being transported). This is followed by injection of 10% calcium gluconate into the subcutaneous tissues. Digital block is usually performed after marking areas of pain. When the block wears off, if pain persists, reinjection is necessary. Even if the block is not complete, it is a briefly painful procedure, and the pain will cease when all of the hydrofluoric acid is neutralized. In large surface area involvement, such as the entire hand, as seen with soaked gloves, treatment consists of placement of a brachial arterial line, followed by 4 to 6 hours of infusion of 10 ml of 10% calcium gluconate in 50 ml of normal saline solution, until the pain is relieved. Repeat as needed until pain is relieved. Multiple infusions are usually necessary.

New treatments may be on the horizon. Hexafluorine has been shown in one study to be effective for cutaneous and eye splash exposure to hydrofluorane.[10,11]

Significant exposures require cardiac monitoring, IV access, and initial and continuing electrolyte monitoring, including calcium, magnesium, and potassium. Watch for ECG changes, such as Q-T prolongation and evidence of hypocalcemia. Intravenous infusion of bicarbonate will enhance renal excretion of fluoride. Hemodialysis may become necessary.[9]

Phosphorus

Phosphorus melts at body temperature and invades deeply into the body tissue. These burns are painful. Care should be taken when copper sulfate is used as an antidote, because copper toxicity can present a danger. The copper will be excreted renally. Hypocalcemia and hyperphosphatemia, with associated myocardial arrhythmias and sudden death can occur.

Treatment. Phosphorus must be washed out of the wound or directly removed using copper solution. Dilute copper sulfate solution (0.5%) deactivates the phosphorus and turns it black to facilitate removal. Adequate urinary output (0.5 ml/kg/hr) must be maintained by administration of fluids or diuretics. ECG monitoring and serial measurement of calcium and phosphate levels should be performed.[12]

REFERENCES

1. Lorette JJ, Wilkinson JA. Alkaline chemical burn to the face requiring full-thickness skin grafting. Ann Emerg Med 17(7):739-741, 1988.
2. Horch R, Spilker G, Stark GB. Phenol burns and intoxications. Burns 20(1): 45-50, 1994.
3. Abbate D, Polito I, Puglisi A, Brecciarohli R, Tanzariella A, Germano D. Dermatosis from resorcinol in tire makers. Br J Ind Med 46(3):212-214, 1989.
4. Schneider MS, Mani MM, Masters FW. Gasoline-induced contact burns. J Burn Care Rehabil 12(2):140-143, 1991.
5. Hunter GA. Chemical burns of the skin after contact with petrol. Br J Plast Surg 21(4):337-341, 1968.
6. Walsh WA, Scarba FJ, Brown RS, Ashcraft KW, Green VA, Holder TM, Amoury RA. Gasoline immersion burn. N Engl J Med 291(16):830-833, 1974.
7. Fujimoto K, Yasuhara N, Kawarada H, Kosaka S, Kawana S. Burns caused by dilute hydrofluoric acid in the bleach. J Nippon Med Sch 69(2):180-184, 2002.
8. Mayer TG, Gross PL. Fatal systemic fluorosis due to hydrofloric acid burns. Ann Emerg Med 14(2):149-153, 1985.
9. McIvor M, Cummings C, Mower M, Wenk RE, Lustgarten JA, Baltazar RF. Sudden cardiac death from acute fluoride intoxication; the role of potassium. Ann Emerg Med 16(7):777-781, 1987.

10. Mathieu L, Nehles J, Blomet J, Hall AH. Efficacy of hexafluorine for emergent decontamination of hydrofluoric acid eye and skin splashes. Vet Hum Toxicol 43(5):263-265, 2001.

11. Sheridan RL, Ryan CM, Quinby WC Jr, Blair J, Tompkins RG, Burke JF. Emergency management of major hydrofluoric acid exposures. Burns 21(1):62-64, 1995.

12. Davis KG. Acute management of white phosphorus burn. Mil Med 167(1):83-84, 2002.

13. Lin CH, Yang JY. Chemical burns with renal integration and multiple organ failure. Burns 18(2):162-166, 1992.

14. Artz CP, Gibson T. Management of burns. Mil Med 141(10):673-679, 1976.

11 ▪ Pediatric Burn Management

INCIDENCE/EPIDEMIOLOGY

Each year approximately 40,000 children age 14 and under are injured in fires in the home. It has been estimated that in 1999, 615 children age 14 and under died as a result of fire and burn-related injury; nearly 60% of these children were under 4 years old. Almost 70% of deaths in children are from inhalation of smoke and/or toxic gases; thermal injury is responsible for the remaining 30%. In 2000 it is estimated that 99,630 children age 14 and under were treated in an ER for burn-related injuries. Of these, 61,370 were thermal burns, 26,110 were scald burns, 6850 were chemical burns, and 2770 were electrical burns. Of those children aged 4 and under hospitalized for burn injuries, it is estimated that 65% are treated for scald burns and 20% for contact burns.[1-4]

After general trauma, fires and burn injuries are the second leading cause of death in children. Fortunately, survival rates have improved in this population over the years. Current management of pediatric burn injuries affords the patient, with an otherwise uncomplicated 90% to 95% burn injury, a 50% chance of survival or better.[5] The mortality rate increases significantly with smoke inhalation injury.

The overall improvement in mortality and outcome can be attributed to multiple factors, including early and aggressive resuscitation, respiratory care and treatment of inhalation injury, control of infection, early burn excision and grafting, and treatment of the hypermetabolic response to trauma.[6]

MONETARY IMPACT

The estimated annual cost of burn deaths and injuries for children age 14 and under is $1.2 billion. Injuries to children 4 and under account for more than $550 million.

Every dollar spent on a smoke alarm can save $69 in fire-related deaths.[1]

The estimated annual cost of scald-related deaths and injuries among children 14 and under is $2.1 billion. Injuries to children age 4 and under account for $1.3 billion, or more than 60% of these costs.[2]

UNIQUE PATIENT POPULATION

Pediatric patients are not just little adults—this is a unique patient population with unique challenges and responses. A child's skin is thinner than an adult's skin; thus it is less capable of protecting the body from thermal injury. The same heat exposure to a child will create a more severe burn injury than in an adult. Children's injuries are likely to be deeper and complicated by contracture and hypertrophic scarring. Secondary disfigurement often exceeds the damage of the original burn wound.[7]

RESUSCITATION

Key issues in pediatric trauma are:
- Airway
- Access
- Ambient temperature

As with adults, a pediatric patient is a trauma patient and needs to be viewed as such. Advanced trauma life support (ATLS) protocols still need to be applied.

Airway

Inhalation injury, with the attendant infection, and pulmonary failure, is a primary determinant of mortality in the thermally injured child. Definitive diagnosis of inhalation injury is by bronchoscopy. The smaller opening of a pediatric airway predisposes it to obstruction. A 1-mm increase in tissue thickness of a 4-mm diameter pediatric trachea results in a 16-fold increase in resistance and a 75% reduction of cross-sectional area. Comparably, it would increase the airway resistance only threefold and reduce the airway area by 44% in an adult.[8]

Hyperextension of the neck is contraindicated in a pediatric patient. Direct laryngoscopy is necessary to examine the larynx and cords for soot or edema. Use a straight blade in children less than 6 years old. A rule of thumb is to use an endotracheal tube the diameter of the child's unburned small finger. We typically use an uncuffed endotracheal tube.

Access

Children with large burn injuries may require two large-vessel access points. Central-vein canalization can be difficult. Femoral or saphenous veins may be the best routes for large-vein access, with a surgical cutdown if necessary. If needed, intraosseous access can be obtained.

Hypovolemic shock may present quickly in pediatric burn victims. This is especially true of infants, as their losses are proportionately larger. For example, 20% total burned surface area (TBSA) in a 10-kg child causes an evaporative loss of 475 ml, or 60% of the circulating volume. The same burn in a 70-kg adult would result in a loss of 1.1 L, or only 20% of the patient's circulating volume.

Ambient Temperature

Infants and toddlers, with their increased surface-to-volume ratio, less insulating fat, and lower muscle mass (for shivering), are prone to hypothermia.

Make an effort to reduce heat loss. Ambient temperature should be 82° to 90° F (28° to 32° C). Bathing and/or showering should be done quickly, and any unnecessary exposure should be avoided.

Surface Area Calculations

The most accurate mapping of the burn wound is after the washing off any loose tissue, soot, or dirt. Children have a larger surface area per unit weight. Infants have a larger surface area of the head, with less surface area on the extremities as compared with adults. Thus the "Rule of nines" must be modified for calculation of TBSA in pediatric patients (see p. 17).

In a child under 1 year of age, the head is approximately 19% of the body mass, while the extremities account for 13% each. A useful rule of thumb is this: For each year over 1, subtract 1% from the head and add 0.5% to each lower extremity. Another useful rule of thumb for estimating burn size: The palmar surface of the child's hand is approximately 1%. One can use this clinically for nonuniform areas.

The Berkow table and the Lund/Browder body chart (see p. 18 or p. i) are the most accurate, and should be used for definitive documentation and calculation of TBSA.

Resuscitation Formulas: Modified Parkland

The Parkland formula is modified in pediatric patients by adding maintenance fluid, to the resuscitation fluid volume, as follows:

$$4 \text{ ml LR} \times \text{kg} \times \%\text{TBSA} + \text{Maintenance fluid} =$$
$$\text{Amount to be given in first 24-hr period}$$

Method for Calculating Maintenance Fluid

First 10 kg	100 ml/kg
Second 10 kg	50 ml/kg
Every kilogram above 20 kg	20 ml/kg

For example, a 30-kg patient's calculation would be 100×10 (for the first 10 kg) + 50×10 (for the second 10 kg) + 10×20 (for the 10 other kg not yet covered): $1000 + 500 + 200 = 1700$ ml/24 hr = 70 ml/hr for maintenance fluids.

Half of the total fluid is given in the first 8 hours after the burn injury; the other half is given in the next 16 hours. The fluid of choice is lactated Ringer's solution. Infants may require administration of some glucose if the finger stick is <80. In this case go to D_5LR. In the first 8 hours of resuscitation we add 1 ampule of bicarbonate for each liter of lactated Ringer's solution for increased sodium needs. In the third 8-hour period after the burn, we add 1 ampule of SPA to each liter of lactated Ringer's solution.

During the second 24 hours discontinue lactated Ringer's solution or D_5–lactated Ringer's solution if that is what you are using. Start $D_5\frac{1}{2}NS$ at the same rate at which the lactated Ringer's solution was being infused. Adjust the fluid rate titrated to the urine output (1.0 ml/kg/hr).

Remember that these are starting points; the rate should be individualized for each patient. The desired urine output is 1 ml/kg/hr. Because of decreased urine-concentrating capabilities in infants, a Foley catheter is essential so that output can be monitored.[9]

During the second 24 hours, 0.45% NaCl is given as replacement because of the small intravascular volume of children; 5% dextrose is added. If only D_5W is given and the infusion rate is too rapid, hyponatremia and seizure may result.[10] Our fluid of choice is $D_5\frac{1}{2}NS$. Fluid rate is titrated to urine output and perfusion status.

Fluid boluses, when needed, are given in amounts of no more than 25% of the total circulating volume:

Total body volume = 10 ml/kg of body weight

Electrolytes should be monitored for hyponatremia (supplementation may be needed). Watch for hypokalemia. Losses should be replaced as potassium phosphate, not potassium chloride, as hypophosphatemia is frequently observed. As always, if hypokalemia is present, one should evaluate the magnesium level.

Volume overload is to be avoided.

Pediatric Burn Physiology

A child's heart is less compliant, and stroke volumes plateau at relatively low filling pressures. This shifts the Starling curve to the left. Cardiac output depends almost exclusively on heart rate, and the immature heart is more sensitive to volume and pressure overload.

Children are prone to development of edema. Pay particular attention to cerebral edema. Maintain head elevation, especially in the initial 24 to 48 hours after a burn injury. Neurologic assessments must be performed frequently. Pulmonary edema is often caused by hydrostatic pressures, and in the absence of an inhalation injury, is almost diagnostic of fluid overload. Treatment of overhydration includes fluid restriction and diuresis.

Blood loss should be replaced on the second postburn day. The usual amount of blood replacement in a 24-hour period is 10 ml/kg, infused over 3 to 4 hours. Unless there is active blood loss, no more than 15 ml/kg should be given over any 24-hour period. Larger quantities can result in cardiopulmonary congestion or severe hypertension.

Adequacy of Resuscitation

The usual signs of hypovolemia in an adult (tachycardia, hypotension, and decreased urine output) are late signs in a pediatric patient. Children have remarkable cardiopulmonary reserve. They often do not show signs of hypovolemia until more than 25% of their circulating volume is lost, when cardiovascular collapse is imminent. This population frequently develops reflex tachycardia secondary to catecholamine release, even with minimal to moderate stress levels. Smaller body size allows lower vascular pressures to circulate the blood. Therefore systolic pressures of <100 mm Hg are common in children age 5 or younger.

Table 11-1. Normal pediatric vital signs

Age (years)	Heart rate (beats/min)	Systolic BP (mm Hg)	Respirations (breaths/min)
<2	100-160	60	30-40
2-5	80-140	70	20-30
6-12	70-120	80	18-25
>12	60-110	90	16-20

Table 11-2. Glasgow Coma Scale

Adults		Infants/Toddlers	
Eye opening			
Spontaneous	4	Spontaneous	4
To speech	3	To speech	3
To pain	2	To pain	2
None	1	None	1
Verbal response			
Oriented	5	Coos, babbles	5
Confused	4	Irritable, cries	4
Inappropriate words	3	Cries to pain	3
Incomprehensible sounds	2	Moans to pain	2
None	1	None	1
Motor response			
Obeys commands	6	Spontaneous moves	6
Localizes pain	5	Withdraws to touch	5
Withdraws from pain	4	Withdraws to pain	4
Flexion posturing	3	Abnormal flexion	3
Extensor posturing	2	Abnormal extension	2
None	1	None	1

Young children with immature kidneys have less tubular concentrating ability. Urine production may continue despite the presence of hypovolemia.

More reliable indicators include mental clarity, pulse pressures, arterial blood gases, distal extremity color and warmth, capillary refill, and body temperature. More than three abnormalities of these indicators denote that the child is in danger. Table 11-1 summarizes normal pediatric vital signs; Table 11-2 contrasts adult and pediatric Glasgow Coma Scale indicators.

METABOLISM/ NUTRITION

Children under 3 years of age, especially infants under 6 months, have a limited amount of glycogen stored in the liver. This may be rapidly depleted during times of stress. Initiation of protein and lipid catabolism for gluconeogenesis is accelerated. Thus blood glucose should be measured every hour for the first 24 hours after a burn injury to avoid hypoglycemia.

Children are growing, and their metabolic rates are higher than those predicted by adult equations. Major catastrophic illnesses and trauma have been demonstrated to produce transient and permanent changes in growth. In severe burns, growth of nails, hair, and bone may be slowed and usually do not catch up after injury. Children often will refuse to eat anything, much less enough calories for basic energy expenditure and healing. This is most often true in children with >20% TBSA. **NOTE: Do *not* confuse BSA (body surface area) with *TBSA* (total *burned* surface area).**

Galveston Formula

Infants	2100 Kcal/m² BSA + 1000 Kcal/m² *TBSA*
Toddlers	2100 Kcal/m² BSA + 1000 Kcal/m² *TBSA*
School-age children	1800 Kcal/m² BSA + 1300 Kcal/m² *TBSA*
Adolescents	1500 Kcal/m² BSA + 1500 Kcal/m² *TBSA*

Body Surface Area Equation

$$[87(H + W) - 2600] \div 10,000 = \text{Surface in m}^2$$

where H equals height in centimeters and W equals weight in kilograms. (Total ***burned*** surface area is computed by using the charts given in Chapter 3, p. 18.)

Modified Curreri Formula

Infants	BMR + (15 Kcal ÷ %***TBSA***)
Toddlers	BMR + (25 Kcal ÷ %***TBSA***)
School-age children	BMR + (40 Kcal ÷ %***TBSA***)
Adolescents	BMR + (40 Kcal ÷ %***TBSA***)

Basal Metabolic Rate (BMR) Equation

Male =
$$66.5 + (13.7 \times \text{Weight in kg}) + (5 \times \text{Height in cm}) - (6.8 \times \text{Age})$$

Female =
$$65.5 + (9.6 \times \text{Weight in kg}) + (1.7 \times \text{Height in cm}) - (4.7 \times \text{Age})$$

Children will tolerate enteral feedings via gastric or duodenal tube 3 to 6 hours after a burn injury. Avoid hyperosmolar feeds that can cause diarrhea. Work with anesthesia colleagues to minimize the length of preoperative NPO orders.

SCALDING INJURIES

Burns to the neck, shoulder, and thoracic wall in young children are almost always secondary to scalding with hot liquids. Adequate release of neck contractures, are essential in children, owing to the risk of impaired growth and possible micrognathia.[11] Anterior chest scalding injuries usually produce deep second- or third-degree burns. The mammary gland is not usually affected. The mammary gland is an epithelial gland and receives blood supply from posterior to the gland. The burn is typically superficial and not one of breast volume. Treatment is conservative, with release of the soft tissue envelope at puberty to allow future breast development, and later resurfacing with a skin graft or flap.

WOUND CARE

The goal of burn wound care is to preserve function and give the best cosmetic result. Topical antimicrobials should be secured with thick fluffy dressings. Surginet (expandable fishnet) dressings and splints may be helpful. One must watch that children do not eat the topical creams. Bathe wounds at least once a day, inspect for infection, and then redress.

Early excision and grafting can be undertaken.[12,13] Decisions are made on an individual case basis by those with experience and expertise in the management of these wounds.

Rehabilitation is a key element, is started early, and continues throughout the long-term follow-up. When joints are not being exercised, they should be splinted in extension. The hands and neck are most prone to contracture.

RECONSTRUCTION, TIMING, AND OTHER ISSUES

The management of a pediatric burn has changed over the years to one of early excision and coverage. The benefits of this approach include less time in the hospital and fewer episodes of infection.[12] Consider repeated scar release and application of skin grafts during the patient's growth-spurt years.[14]

Although some patients surviving severe burns have lingering disability, most have a satisfying quality of life. Comprehensive burn care that includes experienced multidisciplinary aftercare plays a significant role in the recovery process.[13]

UNIQUE ISSUE IN CHILDREN: ABUSE

Often the burn or scald injury in a child is evidence of neglect or abuse. Unfortunately, this may account for 20% of pediatric burn admissions. Most of these injuries are to children less than 3 years of age and are scald or contact burns. The Child Abuse Prevention and Treatment Act of 1974 requires professionals to report suspected abuse. Do not hesitate to admit the patient to the hospital if there is a question of a dangerous home situation.

Signs Suggesting Abuse

- Child is brought for treatment by an unrelated adult.
- There is an unexplained delay in seeking treatment of >12 hours.
- Parental affect is inappropriate: inattentive to the child, lacking empathy, may appear under the influence of alcohol or drugs.
- A sibling of the patient is blamed for the injury.
- Injury is inconsistent with the description of the circumstances of the injury.
- Injury is inconsistent with the developmental capacity of the patient.
- Prior history of accidental or nonaccidental injury to the patient or siblings.
- Prior history of failure to thrive.
- Historical accounts of the injury differ with each interview.
- Injury localized to the perineum, genitalia, and/or buttocks.
- "Mirror image" injuries to the extremities.
- Inappropriate affect of the child (withdrawn and flat affect).
- Evidence of unrelated injuries (e.g., bruises, scars, welts, fractures).

ELECTRICAL CORD BITES

The most common electrical injury in children occurs when the child bites an electrical cord. Ninety percent of these injuries occur in children under 4 years of age. The incidence is greater in boys than in girls by a ratio of 2:1. This is not a conductive heat injury. Tissue destruction can be extensive. No immediate reconstruction is attempted.

Splinting the commissure with orthodontic appliances is the recommended treatment; the appliances are worn 9 to 12 months. Delayed reconstruction can be performed, if necessary. This treatment modality requires a cooperative patient and parents and frequent monitoring by a prosthodontist. In roughly a fourth of patients there is bleeding from the labial artery, typically 1 to 2 weeks after the injury. Parents should be instructed to apply pressure for several minutes in these cases.

Excision of the burn scar with restoration of the labial musculature can be attempted so as to reduce the number of contractions postoperatively.[15-17] Ventral tongue flaps have also been applied to this problem.[18]

Some will debride and perform definitive repair in the first 2 weeks after the burn injury. This approach is usually not recommended unless the combined loss of commissure and lower lip exceeds the distance of one third of the lip.[19]

TOXIC EPIDERMAL NECROLYSIS SYNDROME

Toxic epidermal necrolysis syndrome (TENS) is an acute inflammatory systemic disease that results in extensive epidermal sloughing (see Chapter 8). The burn unit is the appropriate place for management of these patients because of the need for intensive monitoring, dressing changes, and physical/occupational therapy. Intubation is necessary if the airway is involved. Prevention of wound desiccation and infection are key elements to the survival and functional recovery of these patients. Biologic dressings are used. Enteral feedings are started early. Steroid medications are not used. Antibiotics are given to manage specific foci of infection only.[20-22]

PSYCHOSOCIAL CONSIDERATIONS

Patients may have different priorities for reconstruction than their parents and surgeons. In one study, patients usually desired less reconstruction than parents, especially older children. Adolescents desired cosmetic, as opposed to functional, reconstruction. Most severely burned patients wanted only one procedure. These patients had accepted their appearance more readily than those with less severe burns.[23]

Psychologic support is important to secure the best outcome. Numerous social support groups exist in the local community, nationally, and on the Internet. Family and friends are essential in supporting the patient's long-term treatment and rehabilitation—but they too may need support in coping with the experience.

SAMPLE ADMISSION ORDERS

(Do not write comments—shown here in italics—on the order sheet.)

ADMISSION

To pediatric burn unit

DX

s/p trauma, 30% TBSA burn secondary to house fire.

HEIGHT AND WEIGHT

CONDITION

Critical

VITAL SIGNS

Per routine. [Continuous monitoring of vitals. Record qh; call HO if temp >102.5° F (39° C), p <60 or >100, BP <110 systolic or >160 systolic, pulse ox <90. Strict I&O qh; notify HO if <1.0 ml/kg/hr]. Monitor CVP; record qh.

ALLERGIES

(Document allergies. Watch drug interactions.)

ACTIVITY

Bed rest. Head of bed at a 20-degree angle. *(To minimize cerebral and tracheal edema.)* No pillow for head and neck burns. *(To minimize contractures and damage to ears.)*

NURSING

Per routine. Wound care as per unit protocol. *(See Chapter 4 for examples of such a protocol.)*

DIET

NPO if burn >30%. Enteral feedings with TraumaCal or a similar formula. *(Target feedings of 25 Kcal/kg/day times 2.0 [stress factor].)*

See pp. 122-123 to determine caloric need (goal).

Tube feedings:

½ strength @ 25 ml/hr × 4 hr, then
¾ strength @ 25 ml/hr × 4 hr, then
Full strength @ 25 ml/hr × 4 hr, then
Increase 15 ml/q4h to goal.
Check residuals q4h; hold if >150 ml.

IV FLUIDS

The Parkland formula is modified in pediatric patients by adding maintenance fluid to the resuscitation fluid volume.

4 ml LR × kg × %TBSA + Maintenance fluid =
Amount to be given in first 24-hr period

Give half in the first 8-hr period.
Give half in the next 16-hr period.

Method for calculating maintenance fluid:

First 10 kg	100 ml/kg
Second 10 kg	50 ml/kg
Every kilogram above 20 kg	20 ml/kg

EXAMPLE: A 30-kg patient's calculation would be 100 × 10 (for the first 10 kg) + 50 × 10 (for the second 10 kg) + 10 × 20 (for the 10 other kg not yet covered): 1000 + 500 + 200 = 1700 ml/24 hr. This totals 70 ml/hr for maintenance fluids.

The fluid of choice is lactated Ringer's solution. Infants may require administration of some glucose. In the first 8 hours of resuscitation we add 1 ampule of bicarbonate for each liter of lactated Ringer's solution for increased sodium needs. In the third 8-hour postburn period, we add 1 ampule of salt-poor albumin (SPA).

Note: SPA is a 25% solution. Therefore the calculation is 0.1 ml × kg × %TBSA. If your institution uses only plasmanate (a 5% colloid solution), the calculation for colloid administration is 0.5 ml × kg × %TBSA.

> EXAMPLE: Start IVF LR at ___ ml/hr for ___ hours. Add 1 amp $NaCO_2$ to IVF. (If finger stick is <80, start D_5LR). Then decrease LR to ___ ml/hr for 16 hours. Give 1 unit SPA in each liter of LR starting 16 hours postburn. During the second 24 hours D/C LR (or D_5LR). Start ½ NS at current rate. Adjust fluid rate titrated to urine output (1.0 ml/kg/hr). Follow FS to see whether you need to add D_5.

MEDICATIONS

Topical antibiotics

    Silver sulfadiazine (Silvadene) on body; bacitracin-polymyxin B (Polysporin) on face

    Mycostatin (Nystatin) 200,000 U PO/NGT q8h *(to inhibit bacterial transorption)*

    Tetanus toxoid 0.5 ml IM

    Hypertet 250 U IM *(for patient whose history of immunization is not available)*

    Carafate 1 g PO/NGT q6h *(use for a >20% burn)*

    MVI 10 ml IV qd

Pain medications

    Dilaudid 2 mg IV q4h

    MSO_4 8 mg IV q4h

Other agents

    Heparin 2500 U (weight dependent) SQ q8h

    Codeine 30 mg PO q6h prn *(altered physiology, hyperosmolar fluids cause diarrhea)*

ADDITIONAL ORDERS

If the patient has an eye burn:

Polysporin ophthalmic solution (*double-check that the polysporin solution and/or ointment is the ophthalmic type*)

If the patient has a pulmonary injury:

Aminophyline (*6.0 mg/kg IV load, then 0.5 mg/kg/hr IV*)

Ventolin (*0.5 mg in 2 ml NS via nebulizer q4h and prn*)

Heparin (*4000 U [mix with Ventolin nebulizer in the 2 ml NS] will help to decrease pulmonary casts*)

(*Consider bronchoscopic evaluation.*)

If the patient has no pulmonary injury:

Oxygen per nasal cannula or high-humidity face mask

Chest physical therapy

If the patient has sustained electrical injury:

Complete spine series (*Be sure to visualize C7/T1.*)

Long bone x-ray film series

Urine myoglobin and hemoglobin assay

EXTRA ORDERS

NGT to LCWS flush q2h with 30 ml NS

Daily weight measurement

Bed in 20-degree semi-Fowler's position

Elevate extremities

Foot cradle, splints

Abduct shoulders

Foley to gravity

Decubitus precautions

No pillow for a head/neck burn

VENTILATOR SETTINGS AND PEEP

Preferred ventilator: VDR_4

Initial settings

Ausculatory rate 600

PIP 30-35

2-sec inspiration

2-sec expiration

(If your institution does not have this equipment available, use the following standard ventilator settings. For nonburn patients, usually start on AC-10, V_T of 10-15 ml/kg, 100% FIO_2, 5 PEEP. Burn patients require increased respiratory rate and decreased tidal volume, because contraction from the burn limits chest expansion. Therefore start at AC 15-20, V_T 5-10 ml/kg. Check an ABG in 30 min and make adjustments accordingly.)

Obtain an ABG 30 min after the patient is placed on the ventilator *(And make changes accordingly.)*

ABG/carboxyhemoglobin *(Obtain on admission and prn.)*

ECG *(Obtain on admission and prn.)*

CXR *(Obtain on admission; we usually obtain one on M-F, and prn. A CXR is obtained for patients qd if intubated; assess for infiltrate, tube placement, pneumothorax.)*

LABORATORY TESTS

CBC *(On admission and W.)*

SMA-12 *(On admission and M.)*

SMA-7 *(On admission and M-W-F and prn.)*

PT/PTT *(On admission and prn.)*

Sputum C&S *(On admission and prn.)*

Ca, Mg, Phos *(On admission and biweekly.)*

H&H/electrolytes *(q8h; do this until the patient is stable and then prn.)*

Finger stick blood sugar *(On admission and q4h and prn.)*

Urine 24-hr electrolytes *(On admission.)*

HIV/EtOH/urine drug screen *(On admission.)*

B-HCG *(If patient is female.)*

Sickle cell panel *(If patient is black.)*

Eschar BX *(prn)*

Albumin, prealbumin, transferrin *(qw [on M].)*

CONSULTATIONS
> OT/PT
> Nutrition

OTHER CONSULTATIONS *(prn)*
> *(Consent required for HIV testing, placing central lines, grafting, blood transfusions.)*

REFERENCES

1. Injury facts, fire injury. National Safe Kids Campaign, 2002, pp 1-6. Children's National Medical Center, SafeKids.org.
2. Injury facts, burn injury. National Safe Kids Campaign, 2002, pp 1-5. Children's National Medical Center, SafeKids.org.
3. Child fire casualties. Topical fire research series, vol 1 (17):1-6 US Fire Administration, March 2001 (Rev Dec 2001).
4. Deitch EA, Rutan RL. The challenges of children, the first 48 hours. J Burn Care Rehabil 21(5):424-430, 2000.
5. Sheridan RL, Remensnyder JP, Schnitzer JJ, Schulz JT, Ryan CM, Tompkins RG. Current expectations for survival in pediatric burns. Arch Pediatr Adolesc Med 14(3):245-249, 2000.
6. Herndon DN, Spies M. Modern burn care. Semin Pediatr Surg 10(1):28-31, 2001.
7. Harmel RP Jr, Vane DW, King DR. Burn care in children: Special considerations. Clin Plast Surg 13(1):95-105, 1986.
8. Brietman M. Burn physiology. Scritti Biol 7:395-398, 1932.
9. Merrell S, Saffle JR, Sullivan JJ, Navar PD, Kravitz M, Warden GD. Fluid resuscitation in thermally injured children. Am J Surg 152(6):664-669, 1986.
10. O'Neil CE, Hutsler D, Hildreth MA. Basic nutritional guidelines for pediatric burn patients. J Burn Care Rehabil 10(3):278-284, 1989.
11. Almaguer E, Dillon BT, Parry SW. Facial resurfacing at Shriners Burns Institute: A 16 year experience in young burned patients. J Trauma 25:1081-1082, 1985.
12. Xiao-Wu W, Herndon DN, Spies M, Sanford AP, Wolf SE. Effects of delayed wound excision and grafting in severely burned children. Arch Surg 137(9):1049-1054, 2002.
13. Sheridan RL, Hinson MI, Liang MH, Nackel AF, Schoenfeld DA, Ryan CM, Mulligan JL, Tompkins RG. Long-term outcome of children surviving massive burns. JAMA 283(1):69-73, 2000.
14. Goldberg DP, Kucan JO, Bash D. Reconstruction of the burned foot. Clin Plast Surg 27(1):145-161, 2000.

15. Pensler JM, Rosenthal AM. Reconstruction of the oral commissure after an electrical burn. J Burn Care Rehabil 11(1):50-53, 1990.
16. Silverglade D, Ruberg RL. Nonsurgical management of burns to the lips and commissures. Clin Plast Surg 13(1):87-94, 1986.
17. Leake JE, Curtin JW. Electrical burns of the mouth in children. Clin Plast Surg 11(4):669-683, 1984.
18. Donelan MB. Reconstruction of electrical burns of the oral commissure with a ventral tongue flap. Plast Reconstr Surg 95:(7)1155-1164, 1995.
19. Ortiz-Monasterio F, Factor R. Early definitive treatment of electrical burns of the mouth. Plast Reconstr Surg 65:(2)169-176, 1980.
20. Sheridan RL, Weber JM, Schulz JT, Ryan CM, Low HM, Tompkins RG. Management of severe toxic epidermal necrolysis in children. J Burn Care Rehabil 20(6):497-500, 1999.
21. Spies M, Sanford AP, Aili Lao JF, Wolf SE, Herndon DN. Treatment of extensive toxic epidermal necrolysis in children. Pediatrics 108(5):1162-1168, 2001.
22. Sheridan RL, Schulz JT, Ryan CM, Schnitzer JJ, Lawlor D, Driscoll DN, Donelan MB, Tompkins RG. Long term consequences of toxic epidermal necrolysis in children. Pediatrics 109(1):74-78, 2002.
23. Bjarnason D, Phillips LG, McCoy B, Murphy L, McCauley RL, Desai M, Herndon DN, Robson MC. Reconstructive goals for children with burns: Are our goals the same? J Burn Care Rehabil 13(3):389-390, 1992.
24. Hunt JL, Purdue GF, Pownell PH, Rohrich RJ. Burns: Acute burns, burn surgery, and postburn reconstruction. Selected Readings in Plastic Surgery, vol 1, 8(12):1-37, 1997.
25. Latenser BA, Kowal-Vern A. Paediatric burn rehabilitation. Pediatr Rehabil 5(1):3-10, 2002.

Glossary

ABG	arterial blood gas
ARDS	acute respiratory distress syndrome
BCAA	branched-chain amino acid
BEE	basal energy expenditure
bid	twice per day (*bis in die*)
BMR	basal metabolic rate
BP	blood pressure
BSA	body surface area (not burned surface area)
BUN	blood urea nitrogen
BX	biopsy
CO_2	carbon dioxide
Cr	creatinine
C&S	culture and sensitivity
CVP	central venous pressure
CXR	chest x-ray evaluation
dl	deciliter
DX	diagnosis
EFA	essential fatty acid
ER	emergency room
FENa	fractional excretion of sodium
FFA	free fatty acid
FIo_2	fraction of inspired oxygen (how much oxygen dialed into ventilator to have the patient breathe)
GCS	Glasgow Coma Scale
Hb	hemoglobin
HFV	high-frequency ventilation
HO	house officer

H_2O	water
hr	hour
HX	history
IM	intramuscular
I&O	input and output ("ins and outs")
IV	intravenous
JP	Jackson-Pratt urinary drain
kg	kilogram
LFT	liver function test
LLE	left lower extremity
LR	lactated Ringer's solution
LUE	left upper extremity
μg	microgram
mg	milligram
min	minute
ml	milliliter
M-W-F	Monday-Wednesday-Friday
Na	sodium
NaCl	sodium chloride
NGT	nasogastric tube
NO_2	nitrous oxide (mnemonic: Us = 2, like 2 oxygens)
NO_3	nitric oxide
NPO	nothing by mouth (*nil per os*)
NS	normal saline solution
O_2	oxygen
OT	occupational therapy
P	pulse
PEEP	positive end-expiratory pressure
P_{CO_2}	partial pressure of carbon dioxide
pH	acidity-alkalinity measure
PIP	maximum pressure measured by the ventilation during inspiration
PO	by mouth (*per os*)
P_{O_2}	partial pressure of oxygen
POD	postoperative day #____

PRBC	packed red blood cell
prn	as needed (*pro re nata*)
PT	prothrombin time, physical therapy
PTT	partial thromboplastin time
qd	once every day (*quoque die*)
qh	every hour (*quaque hora*)
qid	four times per day (*quater in die*)
qw	every week
RLE	right lower extremity
RQ	respiratory quotient
RR	respiratory rate
RUE	right upper extremity
SMA-7, SMA-12	Sequential Multiple Analyzer blood chemistry tests
s/p	status post
SPA	salt-poor albumin
SQ	subcutaneously
Svo_2	venous oxygen saturation
TBSA	total burned surface area
tid	three times per day (*ter in die*)
T_{max}	maximum temperature per a given time period (usually 24 hours)
TNL	total nitrogen loss
TX	treatment; therapy
UO	urine output
UUN	urinary urea nitrogen
V/Q	ventilation/perfusion
V_T	tidal volume
WBC	white blood cell (count)

Appendix

MORITZ CONTACT CHART*

A burn is the transfer of heat to tissue. The depth of the injury depends on the intensity of the heat and the duration of the contact to produce a full-thickness burn injury.

Temperature		Time for a
°F	°C	third-degree burn
156		1 sec
150	66	2 sec
149		2 sec
140	60	5 sec
133		15 sec
130	54	30 sec
127		60 sec
125	52	2 min
124		3 min
120	49	10 min

*From Moritz AR, Herriquez FE. Studies of thermal injury. II. The relative importance of time and surface temperature in the causation of cutaneous burns. Am J Pathol 23(d):695-720, 1947.

USEFUL RANGES AND EQUATIONS

CVP	Central venous pressure	1-8	mm Hg
MAP	Mean arterial pressure	75-100	mm Hg
PCWP	Wedge pressure	5-12	mm Hg
CO	Cardiac output	4-6	L/min
CI	Cardiac index	2-4	L/min/m^2
SVR	Systemic vascular resistance	800-1200	dynes $\times$ sec/cm^5
PVR	Peripheral vascular resistance	100-200	dynes $\times$ sec/cm^5
CaO_2	Arteriovenous oxygen content $(SaO_2 \times Hb \times 1.39) + (PaO_2 \times 0.0031)$	16-22	ml O_2/100 ml
CvO_2	Venous oxygen content $(SvO_2 \times Hb \times 1.39) + (PvO_2 \times 0.0031)$	12-17	ml O_2/100 ml
$C(a\text{-}v)O_2$	Arteriovenous oxygen difference $CaO_2 - CvO_2$	3.5-5.5	ml O_2/100 ml
DO_2	Oxygen delivery $CaO_2 \times CO \times 10$	700-1400	ml/min
VO_2	Oxygen consumption $C(a\text{-}v)O_2 \times CO \times 10$	150-300	ml/min
O_2ER	Oxygen extraction ratio $VO_2 \div DO_2$	0.23-0.32	

Index

A

ABCs of resuscitation
   adult, 12-13
   pediatric, 116-117
Acute respiratory distress syndrome
      (ARDS), 75
Admission to burn unit
   adult, 29-33
   pediatric, 127-132
Allograft, 37
American Burn Association criteria
      for referral to burn center,
      inside front cover
Antibiotics, 31, 37, 38, 42, 48-52,
      109
   prophylactic, 74
Antifungal agents, 49, 51
Antioxidants, 64

B

Basal energy expenditure (BEE)
      formula, 58
Beds, 39
Burn classification, 3-4, 109

Burn injury
   chemical, 108-113
   depth of, 3-5
   electrical, 104-107
      cord bites, 125
   fire, 42, 115
   physiologic response to, 6-8
      pediatric, 120
   pathophysiology of, 3-9, 43-45
   zones of, 4-5
Burn injuries, incidence, 1, 115
Burn-related deaths, 1, 42, 100,
      105, 115

C

Calculation of body surface area,
      27-28, inside back cover
   pediatric, 118, 123
Calculation of total burned surface
      area, inside front cover, 14,
      15-25
   Berkow/Lund-Browder chart for,
      25
   pediatric, 122-123

Cardiac abnormalities in electrical burns, 105-106
Catheters, 38
Caustics, 108-109
Chemotherapy, 96-97
Clysis, 47
Coconut Grove nightclub fire, 42
Critical care, 34, 44
Curreri formula, 59

D
Debridement, 28, 35-36, 88
Diabetes mellitus, 97
Diet, 30, 31; *see also* Nutrition
Dietitians, 38
Discharge, 39
Dressings, 28, 50, 90, 124

EF
Edema, 6, 73, 109
Electrolytes, 63
Energy expenditure, 58-59
Enteral feeding formulas, 66-67
Enteral vs. parenteral feedings, 64
Eschar, 43, 45
    "golden period" for excision of, 52
Escharotomy, 46
    chemical, 12
    sites, 26
Evaluation, initial, 10-11
    primary survey and, 11-12
    secondary survey and, 12-14, 27-28

Fluid resuscitation, 12, 30, 61-62, 105, 109
    initial, 10-11
    modified pediatric Parkland formula, 118
    Parkland formula, 14, 30
    pediatric, 120-123

GHIJK
Glasgow Coma Scale, 121
Grafting, 36-37, 46
    in pediatric patients, 124
Hospitalizations from burn injuries, 1, 115
Infection, 42-44, 47, 90
    common pathogens in, 42-43
Inhalation injuries
    pathophysiology of, 73-74
    treatment of, 109
Intubation, 72, 117
Isolation, 47

LMN
Laboratory tests, 33
Metabolic rate, 55
    pediatric, 122, 123
Nikolsky's sign, 100
Nutrition
    caloric and protein needs, 58
    electrolytes, 63
    hypermetabolic state and, 54-57
    pediatric, 122
    vitamins, 63
Nutritional status, 60-61

OPQ

Occupational therapists, 37

Oxygen dissociation curve, 77

Oxygenation; *see* Ventilatory support

Pediatric patients
    abuse, 124-125
    burn incidence, 115
    and monetary impact of burns, 116
    physiology, 120
    resuscitation, 116-121
    vital signs, 121

Peripheral vascular disease, 97

Physical therapists, 38

Psychosocial concerns, 126-127

Presentation notes, 34-36

Psychiatric care, 39, 40

RST

Radiation therapy, 96

Radiographs, diagnostic, 109

Rehabilitation, 39

Respiratory quotient
    and diet, 60

Rule of nines, 16, 17, 118

Sample admission orders
    adult, 29-33
    pediatric, 127-132

Scalds, pediatric, 116, 123

Sepsis, 42

Step-down care, 39

Steroidal agents, 74-75

Stress factors and metabolism, 54-55

Tetanus, 48

Thrombosis, 97

Toxic epidermal necrolysis syndrome (TENS), 99-101, 126

UVW

Ulcers
    decubitus, 88
    leg, 97
    Marjolin's, 87
    and pressure reduction devices, 89

Ventilatory equations, 81-83

Ventilatory support, 32-33, 75-83

Wound care products, 91-95

Wound contamination, 88; *see also* Infection

Wound coverage, 35-36, 37, 46-47, 90
    skin grafts, 36, 46

Wound healing, 85-86, 90

NOTES

NOTES

RULE OF NINES

Body diagram for determining total burned surface area (%TBSA)

Numbers (%) are for anterior only and posterior only.

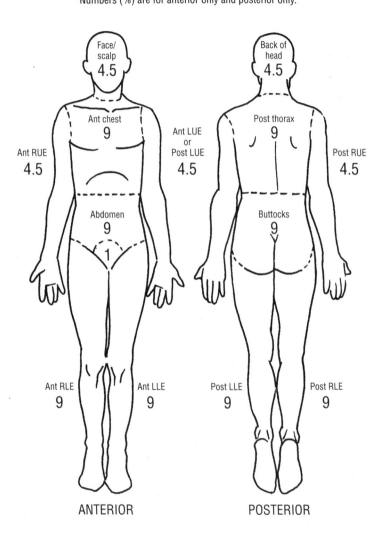

ANTERIOR   POSTERIOR